Acknowledgments:

Thank you....

I0492350

- To my family for loving me as me. I love you all so much!

- To Lori Barklage for being my midwife through out this project.

- To Christina Dietrich, my embodied editor.

- To Kristen Rawson for introducing me to The Neutrality Exercise.

- To all my meditation teachers: Baba Muktananda and Guru Mayi.

- To my mom Kathryn Julia, who set me on a path to self discovery from my conception.

- To everyone and anyone doing any of the work necessary for us humans to find more depth and peace while we share space on this planet together.

An Introduction to The Neutrality Exercise

The Neutrality Exercise is a playful practice that increases our emotional and psychological awareness, and challenges our responses to any topic towards which we choose to apply it. How? By tapping into our imagination through a meditative state.

It can be challenging to remain neutral on a topic in real time. Using our imagination to walk us through various scenarios allows us time and space to process our thoughts and feelings without the pressure of real-time responses. The more we do this, the more ability we have to navigate what could otherwise be reactive situations. We increase our ability to engage in fruitful conversations and establish boundaries that allow everyone to move forward.

It is our experience that doing this exercise repeatedly:
- Decreases our tendency to react.
- Increases our ability to respond.
- Bolsters our ability to establish boundaries.

This workbook is designed to guide you into The Neutrality Exercise as a practice. Our hope is that by doing what is set forth in this workbook, you will establish your own practice. The eventual goal is to apply The Neutrality Exercise to anything you want to challenge your emotional and psychological reactions to. We share this tool with the hope that you apply it toward your own liberation.

***Because The Neutrality Exercise is designed to play with our emotional and psychological responses, be aware that you may be triggered as a result of using it. With that awareness, please be gentle with yourself before, during, and after your practice. Create sufficient space and time to complete the exercise, and be attentive to your feelings. Have your self-care already in place.

4

The more you practice this exercise, the more you will come to find how easily The Neutrality Exercise lends itself to the healing process of using *triggers as medicine.*

Holistic Peer Counseling (HPC)

The Neutrality Exercise is one of several exercises taught as part of a larger Holistic Peer Counseling (HPC) curriculum. Holistic Peer Counseling is Do It Yourself (DIY) technology that teaches the potentially radical perspective that distress patterns need loving attention to heal—and so we practice holding space for our peers' distress patterns. We learn how to be both a client and a counselor so that we can heal ourselves and facilitate healing for others.

Through coming to understand both sides of the counselor/client relationship, we learn tools and distinctions that help us use our personal triggers to catalyze healing—we come to use *triggers as medicine*. The peer counseling dynamic not only keeps the person being counseled in control of their session, it breaks us out of the "I am healer" and "you heal me" mindset. It acknowledges that we all have the ability to give and receive loving attention, and provides opportunities for healing as a result.

Of course, some of us are far better at giving than receiving (and vice versa), and we have myriad programmed responses to receiving attention,. For this as well as many other reasons, the peer counseling process isn't necessarily an easy one to learn; nor is it a quick-fix solution. HPC represents a chance to engage in a challenging, ongoing, life-altering practice that offers literally unimaginable rewards to those who are ready for change.

If you are interested in learning more about HPC, registration is always open at www.holisticpeercounseling.com.

Our textbook is also available on amazon: **Holistic Peer Counseling**.

Getting Started with The Neutrality Exercise

In the beginning, it will serve you to be very intentional about practicing The Neutrality Exercise. As you build up some facility with the tool, you will find you may start practicing in the context of living your life, in real time, almost without noticing.

Because this series is designed for the beginner, we will provide very specific directions. Of course, you can take or leave any directions we may offer.

1—Create the space and time you need to engage in a mindful practice. Sometimes setting a timer can be useful so that you can fully engage in the practice without worrying about using up more time that you have available to you.

2—Practice these exercises in order: (They are laid out in detail on the following pages)
- A Basic Grounding
- The Neutrality Exercise
- Presencing

3—Take some time to use the Introspection pages to integrate what you learned by running through the exercise.

Prior to working The Neutrality Exercise, it is a good idea to get grounded. As such, we are including this Grounding Exercise as a method to calm your body and deepen your awareness. We suggest that you ground prior to each round of The Neutrality Exercise.

Let's begin....

Bringing Attention to Your Breath

You can sit, stand, lie down, or do whatever works best for you. Our aim is to have your body in a state of balance, release, and maybe even in a state of pleasure. If you are seated, your weight should be evenly distributed on your sit bones. If you are standing, keep your weight evenly distributed between your feet. If you are pregnant and lying down, do so on your left side with pillows to support you. If you are not pregnant and want to lie down, do so on your back, perhaps with your knees up and feet on the ground if that is more comfortable for you. Aim for comfort. Aim for relaxation. Aim for pleasure.

Once you are settled, close your eyes or bring them to a soft gaze—whichever brings relaxation to your eyes.

Now, bring your attention to your breathing. Be a witness to it. Notice. Is it fast? Is it slow? Is it deep? Is it shallow? Witness your breathing body like you would calmly witness a new baby discovering its feet for the first time. simply be with it. Feel your inhales and exhales.

You can now become a bit more active with your breath. If you feel a desire to change your breathing at all—perhaps change its rhythm—please do. Maybe you notice you would like to take a deep breath in and let out a sigh. Maybe you feel like doing a little rapid breathing to free it up. Or maybe it's all good just how it is. simply take a moment to experiment with your breath.

Once you have made any desired changes, bring yourself back to the passive witness state again. Be with your breathing. Be with your body. Be with yourself.

Grounding the Body

Bring your attention deep into your lower abdomen, focusing just in front of the spine at the core of your body. Imagine there is a cylindrical tube that attaches this point in your body to the surface of the Earth. You can imagine this tube to be whatever you choose: a hose, a root, a tree trunk, a lava tube, a ray of light. Really see it in your mind's eye and imagine it connecting the center of you with the Earth.

On your next exhale, imagine your tube sinking deeper into the Earth. It falls easily. It gets longer and longer. It falls through all the layers of the Earth. It falls through rock, water, and magma—all the way down to the very center of the Earth. Feel it as the core of your body firmly attaches to the core of Mother Earth. Your bottom is heavy and you feel your connection.

On your next exhale, imagine taking all the energy you don't need right now and sending it down through the tube. Give it to Mother Earth. You don't have to see it or know what it is, simply suggest to yourself that you're letting go of whatever isn't needed right now. It is falling toward the center of the Earth. Where there is tension or pain in your body, relax the area and let it all drain into Mother Earth. This is her compost; she will take it and turn it into fertile soil.

Try to match your breathing with your release: on your inhale, gather all your undesirable energy into a blob of goo and then on your exhale, let it drop down your tube into the Earth. Or you can be more physical about it. On your inhale, stand up and tense your muscles, bringing in and intensifying the energy, and then on your exhale, release all your muscles and fall over or into your seat.

Take some time to practice this on your own for a bit, unguided. During this time, give whatever you want over to Mother Earth through your grounding cord.

Now, take a moment to stop your download and simply feel yourself, feel your grounding cord. Be with what is for a few moments. Bring your attention back to the room slowly. If your eyes are closed, open them slowly. Wiggle your body around a bit. Do what you need to do to bring your awareness back into the room and be present with the people who are here.

In this book we repeatedly offer you two versions of The Neutrality Exercise. One version is designed to take you through different scenarios while looking at a topic. The other is designed to take you through contrasting scenarios related to a topic. Below, you will find general outlines for both versions of The Neutrality Exercise.

As your practice builds, feel free to play with these outlines and create different scenarios for yourself. We give you some space to do that at the end of the book. You really can change any element of the practice to focus on anything in any way you feel will help you better investigate your emotional and psychological responses.

1. The Neutrality Exercise (Single topic: Bubbles)

Imagine you are in the presence of your stated topic. Simply be present with it. Notice how you feel and the thoughts running through my mind being present with it. Be there, be with how you are feeling, and be with the thoughts that come to your mind. (Allow 30-60secs to pass.)

Next, imagine there is a sheet of glass between you and your topic. Notice. Do your feelings change at all while you look at it through a piece of glass? Do your thoughts change? Notice how you feel and the thoughts that come to your mind while looking at your topic through a sheet of glass. (Allow 30-60secs to pass.)

Now, image you are in a huge room—think of a ballroom or a large conference room. Imagine your topic is at the opposite end of the room from you; you can see it, but from far away. Investigate how this feels and what thoughts arise. Did your reaction change at all from the prior scenarios? (Allow 30-60secs to pass.)

Now, imagine you are at the top of a tall tower and the topic is outside the tower, down on the ground. You can barely see it, but you know it is there. See what this feels like and what thoughts come to your mind. (Allow 30-60secs to pass.)

Finally, return to simply being with your topic. Be with your topic and be with how you feel and the thoughts that come to your mind. (Allow 30-60secs to pass.)

2. The Neutrality Exercise (Contrasting topics: Bubbles and no bubbles)

Imagine you are in the presence of your stated topic. Simply be present with it. with it. Notice how you feel and the thoughts running through my mind being present with your topic. Be there, be with how you are feeling, and be with the thoughts that come to your mind. (Allow 30-60secs to pass.)

Next, imagine there is a sheet of glass between you and your topic. Notice. Do your feelings or thoughts change at all while you look at your topic through a piece of glass? Notice how you feel and the thoughts that come to your mind looking at your topic through a sheet of glass. (Allow 30-60secs to pass.)

Now, image you are in a huge room—think of a ballroom or a large conference room. Imagine your topic is at the opposite end of the room from you; you can see it, but from far away. Investigate how this feels and whether your feelings or thoughts change from the prior scenarios. (Allow 30-60secs to pass.)

Now, go back to simply being with your topic. Again, simply be in its presence. Notice how you feel and what thoughts arise being there with it. Be there and be with how you are. (Allow 30-60secs to pass.)

Next, imagine you are in the presence of a contrast to your stated topic. Simply be present with the contrast to your original topic.

Notice how you feel and the thoughts that come to your mind being present with it. Be there and be with how you are. (Allow 30-60secs to pass.)

And then imagine there is a sheet of glass between you and the contrast to your topic. Notice. Do your feelings or thoughts change when you look at it through a piece of glass? Notice how you feel and the thoughts that come to your mind looking at the contrast to your topic through a sheet of glass. (Allow 30-60secs to pass.)

Now, imagine you are in a huge room. Imagine you are at the opposite end of this room from your contrasting topic; you can see it, but from far away. Investigate how this is for you and whether your thoughts or feelings change from the prior scenarios. (Allow 30-60secs to pass.)

Finally, go back to simply being with your topic. Again, simply be in its presence. Maybe notice if your imagination comes to rest more on the original topic or the contrast to it. Notice how you feel and the thoughts that come to your mind being there with whatever you find. Be there and be with how you are. (Allow 30-60secs to pass.)

Finally, go back to just being with your topic. Again, just be in its presence. Maybe notice if your imagination comes to rest more on the original topic or the contrast to it. Notice how you feel and the thoughts that come to your mind being there with whatever you find. Be there and be with how you are. (Allow 30-60secs to pass.)

Presencing

One of the most useful tools from Holistic Peer Counseling is Presencing.

When we are triggered, our attention is no longer in the present moment. Presencing brings our attention back to the present moment so that we can interact with what is happening in the here and now. We find Presencing to be a necessary tool for navigating the trigger-laden world in which we live.

A common Presencing exercise is The Senses Exercise, where we use our senses to bring ourself back to the present moment. We can pay attention to what our eyes are seeing in the space around us. We can use our ears to hear the sounds around us. We can feel the sensations on our skin or in our bodies or pay attention to the smells around us and the tastes in our mouth. Any of these actions can be powerful tools to bring us back to the present moment.

Other methods of Presencing include math problems, jokes, describing something familiar, hopping on one foot, or saying our names over and over. In truth, there are infinite methods of Presencing. If you are new to this practice, start with some of what has been suggested above. Practice often and you will come to better understand the magic of Presencing. Once you acquire some mastery, you will find methods that work best for you.

Before fully stepping away from your practice, take some moments to ponder what you learned from running through The Neutrality Exercise on your specific topic.

You can use these questions below and/or simply express yourself freely in words, patterns, art, etc.

Introspection

- How was that for you?

- What did you learn about yourself?

- Did any of your reactions surprise you?

- How will you incorporate the experience of working The Neutrality Exercise on this topic into your life?

The Entire Practice: Step by Step

1. A Basic Grounding

Bringing Attention to Your Breath

You can sit, stand, lie down, or do whatever works best for you. Our aim is to have your body in a state of balance, release, and maybe even in a state of pleasure. If you are seated, your weight should be evenly distributed on your sit bones. If you are standing, keep your weight evenly distributed between your feet. If you are pregnant and lying down, do so on your left side with pillows to support you. If you are not pregnant and want to lie down, do so on your back, perhaps with your knees up and feet on the ground if that is more comfortable for you. Aim for comfort. Aim for relaxation. Aim for pleasure.

Once you are settled, close your eyes or bring them to a soft gaze—whichever brings relaxation to your eyes.

Now, bring your attention to your breathing. Be a witness to it. Notice. Is it fast? Is it slow? Is it deep? Is it shallow? Witness your breathing body like you would calmly witness a new baby discovering its feet for the first time. simply be with it. Feel your inhales and exhales.

You can now become a bit more active with your breath. If you feel a desire to change your breathing at all—perhaps change its rhythm—please do. Maybe you notice you would like to take a deep breath in and let out a sigh. Maybe you feel like doing a little rapid breathing to free it up. Or maybe it's all good just how it is. simply take a moment to experiment with your breath.

Once you have made any desired changes, bring yourself back to the passive witness state again. Be with your breathing. Be with your body. Be with yourself.

Grounding the Body

Bring your attention deep into your lower abdomen, focusing just in front of the spine at the core of your body. Imagine there is a cylindrical tube that attaches this point in your body to the surface of the Earth. You can imagine this tube to be whatever you choose: a hose, a root, a tree trunk, a lava tube, a ray of light. Really see it in your mind's eye and imagine it connecting the center of you with the Earth.

On your next exhale, imagine your tube sinking deeper into the Earth. It falls easily. It gets longer and longer. It falls through all the layers of the Earth. It falls through rock, water, and magma—all the way down to the very center of the Earth. Feel it as the core of your body firmly attaches to the core of Mother Earth. Your bottom is heavy and you feel your connection.

On your next exhale, imagine taking all the energy you don't need right now and sending it down through the tube. Give it to Mother Earth. You don't have to see it or know what it is, simply suggest to yourself that you're letting go of whatever isn't needed right now. It is falling toward the center of the Earth. Where there is tension or pain in your body, relax the area and let it all drain into Mother Earth. This is her compost; she will take it and turn it into fertile soil.

Try to match your breathing with your release: on your inhale, gather all your undesirable energy into a blob of goo and then on your exhale, let it drop down your tube into the Earth. Or you can be more physical about it. On your inhale, stand up and tense your muscles, bringing in and intensifying the energy, and then on your

exhale, release all your muscles and fall over or into your seat.

Take some time to practice this on your own for a bit, unguided. During this time, give whatever you want over to Mother Earth through your grounding cord.

Now, take a moment to stop your download and simply feel yourself, feel your grounding cord. Be with what is for a few moments. Bring your attention back to the room slowly. If your eyes are closed, open them slowly. Wiggle your body around a bit. Do what you need to do to bring your awareness back into the room and be present with the people who are here.

2. The Neutrality Exercise (A or B)

A. Example 1 (Non-contrasting)

Imagine you are in the presence of your stated topic. Simply be present with it. Notice how you feel and the thoughts running through my mind being present with it. Be there, be with how you are feeling, and be with the thoughts that come to your mind. (Allow 30-60secs to pass.)

Next, imagine there is a sheet of glass between you and your topic. Notice. Do your feelings change at all while you look at it through a piece of glass? Do your thoughts change? Notice how you feel and the thoughts that come to your mind while looking at your topic through a sheet of glass. (Allow 30-60secs to pass.)

Now, image you are in a huge room—think of a ballroom or a large conference room. Imagine your topic is at the opposite end of the room from you; you can see it, but from far away. Investigate how this feels and what thoughts arise. Did your reaction change at all from the prior scenarios? (Allow 30-60secs to pass.)

Now, imagine you are at the top of a tall tower and the topic is outside the tower, down on the ground. You can barely see it, but you know it is there. See what this feels like and what thoughts come to your mind. (Allow 30-60secs to pass.)

Finally, return to simply being with your topic. Be with your topic and be with how you feel and the thoughts that come to your mind. (Allow 30-60secs to pass.)

B. Example 2 (Contrasting)

Imagine you are in the presence of your stated topic. Simply be present with it. with it. Notice how you feel and the thoughts running through my mind being present with your topic. Be there, be with how you are feeling, and be with the thoughts that come to your mind. (Allow 30-60secs to pass.)

Next, imagine there is a sheet of glass between you and your topic. Notice. Do your feelings or thoughts change at all while you look at your topic through a piece of glass? Notice how you feel and the thoughts that come to your mind looking at your topic through a sheet of glass. (Allow 30-60secs to pass.)

Now, image you are in a huge room—think of a ballroom or a large conference room. Imagine your topic is at the opposite end of the room from you; you can see it, but from far away. Investigate how this feels and whether your feelings or thoughts change from the prior scenarios. (Allow 30-60secs to pass.)

Now, go back to simply being with your topic. Again, simply be in its presence. Notice how you feel and what thoughts arise being there with it. Be there and be with how you are. (Allow 30-60secs to pass.)

Next, imagine you are in the presence of a contrast to your stated topic. Simply be present with the contrast to your original topic. Notice how you feel and the thoughts that come to your mind being present with it. Be there and be with how you are. (Allow 30-60secs to pass.)

And then imagine there is a sheet of glass between you and the contrast to your topic. Notice. Do your feelings or thoughts change when you look at it through a piece of glass? Notice how you feel and the thoughts that come to your mind looking at the contrast to your topic through a sheet of glass. (Allow 30-60secs to pass.)

Now, imagine you are in a huge room. Imagine you are at the opposite end of this room from your contrasting topic; you can see it, but from far away. Investigate how this is for you and whether your thoughts or feelings change from the prior scenarios. (Allow 30-60secs to pass.)

Finally, go back to simply being with your topic. Again, simply be in its presence. Maybe notice if your imagination comes to rest more on the original topic or the contrast to it. Notice how you feel and the thoughts that come to your mind being there with whatever you find. Be there and be with how you are. (Allow 30-60secs to pass.)

3. Presence Yourself

Take a moment to bring your awareness back into the present moment. Open your eyes and look around you. See what is in the space with you. Hear the sounds that are around you. Feel the air around you and the body you are living in. You can even pay attention to what you are tasting and smelling. Take some moments to bring your attention to the present moment and away from the topic you just explored.

4. Introspection

Use the following page(s) to write on what you learned about yourself by practicing The Neutrality Exercise. In particular, pay attention to anything you may have learned about your emotional attachments and biases as they relate to the topic.

Questions:

- How was that for you?

- What did you learn about yourself?

- Did any of your reactions surprise you?

- How will you incorporate the experience of working The Neutrality Exercise on this topic into your life?

Topic 1: Bubbles

We want your first round with The Neutrality Exercise to both be unrelated to the general topic of this book and be something that doesn't tend to be very triggering for people. As such, we have chosen: bubbles.

Get yourself settled and let's run through it.

1. A Basic Grounding

Bringing Attention to Your Breath

You can sit, stand, lie down, or do whatever works best for you. Our aim is to have your body in a state of balance, release, and maybe even in a state of pleasure. If you are seated, your weight should be evenly distributed on your sit bones. If you are standing, keep your weight evenly distributed between your feet. If you are pregnant and lying down, do so on your left side with pillows to support you. If you are not pregnant and want to lie down, do so on your back, perhaps with your knees up and feet on the ground if that is more comfortable for you. Aim for comfort. Aim for relaxation. Aim for pleasure.

Once you are settled, close your eyes or bring them to a soft gaze—whichever brings relaxation to your eyes.

Now, bring your attention to your breathing. Be a witness to it. Notice. Is it fast? Is it slow? Is it deep? Is it shallow? Witness your breathing body like you would calmly witness a new baby discovering its feet for the first time. simply be with it. Feel your inhales and exhales.

You can now become a bit more active with your breath. If you feel a

desire to change your breathing at all—perhaps change its rhythm—
please do. Maybe you notice you would like to take a deep breath in
and let out a sigh. Maybe you feel like doing a little rapid breathing
to free it up. Or maybe it's all good just how it is. simply take a
moment to experiment with your breath.

Once you have made any desired changes, bring yourself back to the
passive witness state again. Be with your breathing. Be with your
body. Be with yourself.

Grounding the Body

Bring your attention deep into your lower abdomen, focusing just in
front of the spine at the core of your body. Imagine there is a
cylindrical tube that attaches this point in your body to the surface
of the Earth. You can imagine this tube to be whatever you choose: a
hose, a root, a tree trunk, a lava tube, a ray of light. Really see it in
your mind's eye and imagine it connecting the center of you with the
Earth.

On your next exhale, imagine your tube sinking deeper into the
Earth. It falls easily. It gets longer and longer. It falls through all the
layers of the Earth. It falls through rock, water, and magma—all the
way down to the very center of the Earth. Feel it as the core of your
body firmly attaches to the core of Mother Earth. Your bottom is
heavy and you feel your connection.

On your next exhale, imagine taking all the energy you don't need
right now and sending it down through the tube. Give it to Mother
Earth. You don't have to see it or know what it is, simply suggest to
yourself that you're letting go of whatever isn't needed right now. It
is falling toward the center of the Earth. Where there is tension or
pain in your body, relax the area and let it all drain into Mother
Earth. This is her compost; she will take it and turn it into fertile soil.

Try to match your breathing with your release: on your inhale, gather all your undesirable energy into a blob of goo and then on your exhale, let it drop down your tube into the Earth. Or you can be more physical about it. On your inhale, stand up and tense your muscles, bringing in and intensifying the energy, and then on your exhale, release all your muscles and fall over or into your seat.

Take some time to practice this on your own for a bit, unguided. During this time, give whatever you want over to Mother Earth through your grounding cord.

Now, take a moment to stop your download and simply feel yourself, feel your grounding cord. Be with what is for a few moments. Bring your attention back to the room slowly. If your eyes are closed, open them slowly. Wiggle your body around a bit. Do what you need to do to bring your awareness back into the room and be present with the people who are here.

2. The Neutrality Exercise: Bubbles

Imagine you are in the presence of bubbles. Simply be there with them. Notice how it is for you to be there with bubbles. Be there with them; be with how you are feeling and the thoughts that come to your mind. (Allow 30–60 seconds to pass.)

Next, imagine there is a sheet of glass between you and bubbles. Notice. Do your feelings change at all while you look at bubbles through a sheet of glass? Do your thoughts change? Notice how you feel and the thoughts that come to your mind being with bubbles while having a sheet of glass between you and them. (Allow 30–60 seconds to pass.)

Now, imagine you are in a huge room—think of a ballroom or large conference room. Imagine the bubbles are at the opposite end of the room from you; you can see them, but from far away. Investigate how this feels and whether your feelings or thoughts change from the prior scenario. (Allow 30–60 seconds to pass.)

And now, imagine you are at the top of a tall tower and the bubbles are outside the tower, down on the ground. What does it feel like and what thoughts come to your mind when you look at bubbles far down below you? (Allow 30–60 seconds to pass.)

Finally, return to simply being with bubbles. Be with the bubbles and be with how you feel and the thoughts that come to your mind being there with them. (Allow 30–60 seconds to pass.)

3. Presence Yourself

Before you step away completely, take a moment to bring your awareness back into the present moment. Open your eyes and look around you. See what is in the space with you. Hear the sounds that are around you. Feel the air around you and the body you are living in. You can even pay attention to what you are tasting and smelling. Take some moments to bring your attention to the present moment and away from the topic you simply explored.

4. Introspection

How was that for you?

What did you learn about yourself?

Did any of your reactions surprise you?

How will you bring the experience of working The Neutrality Exercise on this topic into your life?

The Neutrality Exercise Workbook for Birth Doulas

Topic 2: Pregnancy

1. A Basic Grounding

Bringing Attention to Your Breath

You can sit, stand, lie down, or do whatever works best for you. Our aim is to have your body in a state of balance, release, and maybe even in a state of pleasure. If you are seated, your weight should be evenly distributed on your sit bones. If you are standing, keep your weight evenly distributed between your feet. If you are pregnant and lying down, do so on your left side with pillows to support you. If you are not pregnant and want to lie down, do so on your back, perhaps with your knees up and feet on the ground if that is more comfortable for you. Aim for comfort. Aim for relaxation. Aim for pleasure.

Once you are settled, close your eyes or bring them to a soft gaze—whichever brings relaxation to your eyes.

Now, bring your attention to your breathing. Be a witness to it. Notice. Is it fast? Is it slow? Is it deep? Is it shallow? Witness your breathing body like you would calmly witness a new baby discovering its feet for the first time. simply be with it. Feel your inhales and exhales.

You can now become a bit more active with your breath. If you feel a desire to change your breathing at all—perhaps change its rhythm—please do. Maybe you notice you would like to take a deep breath in and let out a sigh. Maybe you feel like doing a little rapid breathing to free it up. Or maybe it's all good just how it is. simply take a moment to experiment with your breath.

Once you have made any desired changes, bring yourself back to the passive witness state again. Be with your breathing. Be with your body. Be with yourself.

Grounding the Body

Bring your attention deep into your lower abdomen, focusing simply in front of the spine at the core of your body. Imagine there is a cylindrical tube that attaches this point in your body to the surface of the Earth. You can imagine this tube to be whatever you choose: a hose, a root, a tree trunk, a lava tube, a ray of light. Really see it in your mind's eye and imagine it connecting the center of you with the Earth.

On your next exhale, imagine your tube sinking deeper into the Earth. It falls easily. It gets longer and longer. It falls through all the layers of the Earth. It falls through rock, water, and magma—all the way down to the very center of the Earth. Feel it as the core of your body firmly attaches to the core of Mother Earth. Your bottom is heavy and you feel your connection.

On your next exhale, imagine taking all the energy you don't need right now and sending it down through the tube. Give it to Mother Earth. You don't have to see it or know what it is, simply suggest to yourself that you're letting go of whatever isn't needed right now. It is falling toward the center of the Earth. Where there is tension or pain in your body, relax the area and let it all drain into Mother Earth. This is her compost; she will take it and turn it into fertile soil.

Try to match your breathing with your release: on your inhale, gather all your undesirable energy into a blob of goo and then on your exhale, let it drop down your tube into the Earth. Or you can be more physical about it. On your inhale, stand up and tense your muscles, bringing in and intensifying the energy, and then on your

exhale, release all your muscles and fall over or into your seat.

Take some time to practice this on your own for a bit, unguided. During this time, give whatever you want over to Mother Earth through your grounding cord.

Now, take a moment to stop your download and simply feel yourself, feel your grounding cord. Be with what is for a few moments. Bring your attention back to the room slowly. If your eyes are closed, open them slowly. Wiggle your body around a bit. Do what you need to do to bring your awareness back into the room and be present with the people who are here.

2. The Neutrality Exercise: Pregnancy

Take a moment to contemplate pregnancy. Really imagine what that word means to you: pregnancy. Notice how you feel and the thoughts that run through your mind as you contemplate pregnancy. Be there, be with how you are feeling, and be with the thoughts that arise in your mind. (Allow 30–60 seconds to pass.)

Next, imagine there is a sheet of glass between you and whatever your mind lands on as you contemplate pregnancy. Notice. Do your feelings change at all while you look through a sheet of glass at whatever comes to your mind as you contemplate pregnancy? Do your thoughts change? Notice how you feel and the thoughts that come to your mind having a sheet of glass between you and whatever your mind lands on as you contemplate pregnancy. (Allow 30–60 seconds to pass.)

Now, image you are in a huge room—think of a ballroom or a large conference room. Whatever your mind lands on as you contemplate pregnancy is at one end of the room and you are at the other.

Investigate how this feels and what thoughts arise in your mind as you look at whatever comes to your mind as you contemplate pregnancy on the opposite end of a large room from you. Did your reaction change at all from the prior scenarios? (Allow 30–60 seconds to pass.)

And now, imagine you are at the top of a tall tower, and whatever your mind lands on as you contemplate pregnancy is outside the tower, down on the ground far below you. See what this feels like and notice the thoughts that come to your mind as you look far below you at whatever comes to your mind as you contemplate pregnancy. (Allow 30–60 seconds to pass.)

Finally, return to simply being with the word pregnancy again. Be with how you feel and the thoughts that come to your mind. (Allow 30–60 seconds to pass.)

3. Presence Yourself

Before you step away completely, take a moment to bring your awareness back into the present moment. Open your eyes and look around you. See what is in the space with you. Hear the sounds that are around you. Feel the air around you and the body you are living in. You can even pay attention to what you are tasting and smelling. Take some moments to bring your attention to the present moment and away from the topic you just explored.

4. Introspection

How was that for you?

What did you learn about yourself?

Did any of your reactions surprise you?

How will you bring the experience of working The Neutrality Exercise on this topic into your life?

The Neutrality Exercise Workbook for Birth Doulas

Topic 3: Labor

1. A Basic Grounding

Bringing Attention to Your Breath

You can sit, stand, lie down, or do whatever works best for you. Our aim is to have your body in a state of balance, release, and maybe even in a state of pleasure. If you are seated, your weight should be evenly distributed on your sit bones. If you are standing, keep your weight evenly distributed between your feet. If you are pregnant and lying down, do so on your left side with pillows to support you. If you are not pregnant and want to lie down, do so on your back, perhaps with your knees up and feet on the ground if that is more comfortable for you. Aim for comfort. Aim for relaxation. Aim for pleasure.

Once you are settled, close your eyes or bring them to a soft gaze—whichever brings relaxation to your eyes.

Now, bring your attention to your breathing. Be a witness to it. Notice. Is it fast? Is it slow? Is it deep? Is it shallow? Witness your breathing body like you would calmly witness a new baby discovering its feet for the first time. simply be with it. Feel your inhales and exhales.

You can now become a bit more active with your breath. If you feel a desire to change your breathing at all—perhaps change its rhythm—please do. Maybe you notice you would like to take a deep breath in and let out a sigh. Maybe you feel like doing a little rapid breathing to free it up. Or maybe it's all good just how it is. simply take a moment to experiment with your breath.

Once you have made any desired changes, bring yourself back to the passive witness state again. Be with your breathing. Be with your body. Be with yourself.

Grounding the Body

Bring your attention deep into your lower abdomen, focusing simply in front of the spine at the core of your body. Imagine there is a cylindrical tube that attaches this point in your body to the surface of the Earth. You can imagine this tube to be whatever you choose: a hose, a root, a tree trunk, a lava tube, a ray of light. Really see it in your mind's eye and imagine it connecting the center of you with the Earth.

On your next exhale, imagine your tube sinking deeper into the Earth. It falls easily. It gets longer and longer. It falls through all the layers of the Earth. It falls through rock, water, and magma—all the way down to the very center of the Earth. Feel it as the core of your body firmly attaches to the core of Mother Earth. Your bottom is heavy and you feel your connection.

On your next exhale, imagine taking all the energy you don't need right now and sending it down through the tube. Give it to Mother Earth. You don't have to see it or know what it is, simply suggest to yourself that you're letting go of whatever isn't needed right now. It is falling toward the center of the Earth. Where there is tension or pain in your body, relax the area and let it all drain into Mother Earth. This is her compost; she will take it and turn it into fertile soil.

Try to match your breathing with your release: on your inhale, gather all your undesirable energy into a blob of goo and then on your exhale, let it drop down your tube into the Earth. Or you can be more physical about it. On your inhale, stand up and tense your muscles, bringing in and intensifying the energy, and then on your

exhale, release all your muscles and fall over or into your seat.

Take some time to practice this on your own for a bit, unguided. During this time, give whatever you want over to Mother Earth through your grounding cord.

Now, take a moment to stop your download and simply feel yourself, feel your grounding cord. Be with what is for a few moments. Bring your attention back to the room slowly. If your eyes are closed, open them slowly. Wiggle your body around a bit. Do what you need to do to bring your awareness back into the room and be present with the people who are here.

2. The Neutrality Exercise: Labor

Take a moment to contemplate labor. Really imagine what that word means to you: labor. Notice how you feel and the thoughts that run through your mind as you contemplate what labor means to you. Be there, be with how you are feeling, and be with the thoughts that arise in your mind. (Allow 30-60secs to pass.)

Next, imagine there is a sheet of glass between you and whatever your mind lands on as you contemplate labor. Notice. Do your feelings change when you look through a sheet of glass at what comes to your mind as you contemplate labor? Do your thoughts change? Notice how you feel and the thoughts that come to your mind having a sheet of glass between you and whatever your mind lands on as you contemplate labor. (Allow 30-60secs to pass.)

Now, image you are in a huge room—think of a ballroom or large conference room. Whatever your mind lands on as you contemplate labor is at one end of the room and you are at the other. Investigate how this feels and the thoughts that come to your mind. Did your reaction change at all from the prior scenarios? (Allow 30-60secs to pass.)

And now, imagine you are at the top of a tall tower and whatever your mind lands on as you contemplate labor is outside the tower, down on the ground far below you. See what this feels like and notice the thoughts that come to your mind as you look far below you at whatever comes to your mind as you contemplate labor. (Allow 30-60secs to pass.)

Finally, return to simply being with the word labor again. Be with how you feel and the thoughts that come to your mind. (Allow 30-60secs to pass.)

3. Presence Yourself

Before you step away completely, take a moment to bring your awareness back into the present moment. Open your eyes and look around you. See what is in the space with you. Hear the sounds that are around you. Feel the air around you and the body you are living in. You can even pay attention to what you are tasting and smelling. Take some moments to bring your attention to the present moment and away from the topic you just explored.

4. Introspection

How was that for you?

What did you learn about yourself?

Did any of your reactions surprise you?

How will you bring the experience of working The Neutrality Exercise on this topic into your life?

The Neutrality Exercise Workbook for Birth Doulas

Topic 4: Birth

1. A Basic Grounding

Bringing Attention to Your Breath

You can sit, stand, lie down, or do whatever works best for you. Our aim is to have your body in a state of balance, release, and maybe even in a state of pleasure. If you are seated, your weight should be evenly distributed on your sit bones. If you are standing, keep your weight evenly distributed between your feet. If you are pregnant and lying down, do so on your left side with pillows to support you. If you are not pregnant and want to lie down, do so on your back, perhaps with your knees up and feet on the ground if that is more comfortable for you. Aim for comfort. Aim for relaxation. Aim for pleasure.

Once you are settled, close your eyes or bring them to a soft gaze—whichever brings relaxation to your eyes.

Now, bring your attention to your breathing. Be a witness to it. Notice. Is it fast? Is it slow? Is it deep? Is it shallow? Witness your breathing body like you would calmly witness a new baby discovering its feet for the first time. simply be with it. Feel your inhales and exhales.

You can now become a bit more active with your breath. If you feel a desire to change your breathing at all—perhaps change its rhythm—please do. Maybe you notice you would like to take a deep breath in and let out a sigh. Maybe you feel like doing a little rapid breathing to free it up. Or maybe it's all good just how it is. simply take a moment to experiment with your breath.

Once you have made any desired changes, bring yourself back to the passive witness state again. Be with your breathing. Be with your body. Be with yourself.

Grounding the Body

Bring your attention deep into your lower abdomen, focusing simply in front of the spine at the core of your body. Imagine there is a cylindrical tube that attaches this point in your body to the surface of the Earth. You can imagine this tube to be whatever you choose: a hose, a root, a tree trunk, a lava tube, a ray of light. Really see it in your mind's eye and imagine it connecting the center of you with the Earth.

On your next exhale, imagine your tube sinking deeper into the Earth. It falls easily. It gets longer and longer. It falls through all the layers of the Earth. It falls through rock, water, and magma—all the way down to the very center of the Earth. Feel it as the core of your body firmly attaches to the core of Mother Earth. Your bottom is heavy and you feel your connection.

On your next exhale, imagine taking all the energy you don't need right now and sending it down through the tube. Give it to Mother Earth. You don't have to see it or know what it is, simply suggest to yourself that you're letting go of whatever isn't needed right now. It is falling toward the center of the Earth. Where there is tension or pain in your body, relax the area and let it all drain into Mother Earth. This is her compost; she will take it and turn it into fertile soil.

Try to match your breathing with your release: on your inhale, gather all your undesirable energy into a blob of goo and then on your exhale, let it drop down your tube into the Earth. Or you can be more physical about it. On your inhale, stand up and tense your muscles, bringing in and intensifying the energy, and then on your

exhale, release all your muscles and fall over or into your seat.

Take some time to practice this on your own for a bit, unguided. During this time, give whatever you want over to Mother Earth through your grounding cord.

Now, take a moment to stop your download and simply feel yourself, feel your grounding cord. Be with what is for a few moments. Bring your attention back to the room slowly. If your eyes are closed, open them slowly. Wiggle your body around a bit. Do what you need to do to bring your awareness back into the room and be present with the people who are here.

2. The Neutrality Exercise: Birth

Take a moment to contemplate birth. Really imagine what that word means to you: birth. Notice how you feel and the thoughts that run through your mind as you contemplate birth. Be there, be with how you are feeling, and be with the thoughts that arise in your mind. (Allow 30–60 seconds to pass.)

Next, imagine there is a sheet of glass between you and whatever your mind lands on as you contemplate birth. Notice. Do your feelings change at all while you look through a sheet of glass at whatever comes to your mind as you contemplate birth? Do your thoughts change? Notice how you feel and the thoughts that come to your mind having a sheet of glass between you and whatever your mind lands on as you contemplate birth. (Allow 30–60 seconds to pass.)

Now, image you are in a huge room—think of a ballroom or a large conference room. Whatever your mind lands on as you contemplate birth is at one end of the room and you are at the other. Investigate how this feels. Notice the thoughts that arise in your mind. Did your reaction change at all from the prior scenarios? (Allow 30–60 seconds to pass.)

And now, imagine you are at the top of a tall tower, and whatever your mind lands on as you contemplate birth is outside the tower, down on the ground far below you. See what this feels like and notice the thoughts that come to your mind as you look far below you at whatever comes to your mind as you contemplate birth. (Allow 30–60 seconds to pass.)

Finally, return to simply being with the word birth again. Be with how you feel and the thoughts that come to your mind. (Allow 30–60 seconds to pass.)

3. Presence Yourself

Before you step away completely, take a moment to bring your awareness back into the present moment. Open your eyes and look around you. See what is in the space with you. Hear the sounds that are around you. Feel the air around you and the body you are living in. You can even pay attention to what you are tasting and smelling. Take some moments to bring your attention to the present moment and away from the topic you just explored.

4. Introspection

How was that for you?

What did you learn about yourself?

Did any of your reactions surprise you?

How will you bring the experience of working The Neutrality Exercise on this topic into your life?

The Neutrality Exercise Workbook for Birth Doulas

Topic 5: Death

1. A Basic Grounding

Bringing Attention to Your Breath

You can sit, stand, lie down, or do whatever works best for you. Our aim is to have your body in a state of balance, release, and maybe even in a state of pleasure. If you are seated, your weight should be evenly distributed on your sit bones. If you are standing, keep your weight evenly distributed between your feet. If you are pregnant and lying down, do so on your left side with pillows to support you. If you are not pregnant and want to lie down, do so on your back, perhaps with your knees up and feet on the ground if that is more comfortable for you. Aim for comfort. Aim for relaxation. Aim for pleasure.

Once you are settled, close your eyes or bring them to a soft gaze—whichever brings relaxation to your eyes.

Now, bring your attention to your breathing. Be a witness to it. Notice. Is it fast? Is it slow? Is it deep? Is it shallow? Witness your breathing body like you would calmly witness a new baby discovering its feet for the first time. simply be with it. Feel your inhales and exhales.

You can now become a bit more active with your breath. If you feel a desire to change your breathing at all—perhaps change its rhythm—please do. Maybe you notice you would like to take a deep breath in and let out a sigh. Maybe you feel like doing a little rapid breathing to free it up. Or maybe it's all good just how it is. simply take a moment to experiment with your breath.

Once you have made any desired changes, bring yourself back to the passive witness state again. Be with your breathing. Be with your body. Be with yourself.

Grounding the Body

Bring your attention deep into your lower abdomen, focusing simply in front of the spine at the core of your body. Imagine there is a cylindrical tube that attaches this point in your body to the surface of the Earth. You can imagine this tube to be whatever you choose: a hose, a root, a tree trunk, a lava tube, a ray of light. Really see it in your mind's eye and imagine it connecting the center of you with the Earth.

On your next exhale, imagine your tube sinking deeper into the Earth. It falls easily. It gets longer and longer. It falls through all the layers of the Earth. It falls through rock, water, and magma—all the way down to the very center of the Earth. Feel it as the core of your body firmly attaches to the core of Mother Earth. Your bottom is heavy and you feel your connection.

On your next exhale, imagine taking all the energy you don't need right now and sending it down through the tube. Give it to Mother Earth. You don't have to see it or know what it is, simply suggest to yourself that you're letting go of whatever isn't needed right now. It is falling toward the center of the Earth. Where there is tension or pain in your body, relax the area and let it all drain into Mother Earth. This is her compost; she will take it and turn it into fertile soil.

Try to match your breathing with your release: on your inhale, gather all your undesirable energy into a blob of goo and then on your exhale, let it drop down your tube into the Earth. Or you can be more physical about it. On your inhale, stand up and tense your muscles, bringing in and intensifying the energy, and then on your

exhale, release all your muscles and fall over or into your seat.

Take some time to practice this on your own for a bit, unguided. During this time, give whatever you want over to Mother Earth through your grounding cord.

Now, take a moment to stop your download and simply feel yourself, feel your grounding cord. Be with what is for a few moments. Bring your attention back to the room slowly. If your eyes are closed, open them slowly. Wiggle your body around a bit. Do what you need to do to bring your awareness back into the room and be present with the people who are here.

2. The Neutrality Exercise: Death

Take a moment to contemplate death. Whatever your mind lands on related to death, take a moment to be with it. Notice how you feel and the thoughts that run through your mind being present with whatever your mind lands on as you contemplate death. Be there, be with how you feel, and be with the thoughts that come to your mind. (Allow 30–60 seconds to pass.)

Next, imagine there is a sheet of glass between you and whatever your mind lands on as you contemplate death. Notice. Do your feelings change at all while you look at it through a sheet of glass? Do your thoughts change? Notice how you feel and the thoughts that come to your mind having a sheet of glass between you and whatever your mind lands on as you contemplate death. (Allow 30–60 seconds to pass.)

Now, image you are in a huge room—think of a ballroom or a large conference room. Imagine whatever your mind lands on as you contemplate death is at the opposite end of the room from you.

Investigate how this feels and what thoughts arise. Does your reaction change at all from the prior scenarios? (Allow 30–60 seconds to pass.)

And now, imagine you are at the top of a tall tower, and whatever your mind lands on as you contemplate death is outside the tower, down on the ground. You can barely see it, but you know it is there. See what this feels like and what thoughts come to your mind. (Allow 30–60 seconds to pass.)

Finally, return to simply being with whatever comes to your mind as you contemplate death, again. Be with how you feel and the thoughts that come to your mind. (Allow 30–60 seconds to pass.)

3. Presence Yourself

Before you step away completely, take a moment to bring your awareness back into the present moment. Open your eyes and look around you. See what is in the space with you. Hear the sounds that are around you. Feel the air around you and the body you are living in. You can even pay attention to what you are tasting and smelling. Take some moments to bring your attention to the present moment and away from the topic you just explored.

4. Introspection

How was that for you?

What did you learn about yourself?

Did any of your reactions surprise you?

How will you bring the experience of working The Neutrality Exercise on this topic into your life?

The Neutrality Exercise Workbook for Birth Doulas

Topic 6: Bodily Fluids

1. A Basic Grounding

Bringing Attention to Your Breath

You can sit, stand, lie down, or do whatever works best for you. Our aim is to have your body in a state of balance, release, and maybe even in a state of pleasure. If you are seated, your weight should be evenly distributed on your sit bones. If you are standing, keep your weight evenly distributed between your feet. If you are pregnant and lying down, do so on your left side with pillows to support you. If you are not pregnant and want to lie down, do so on your back, perhaps with your knees up and feet on the ground if that is more comfortable for you. Aim for comfort. Aim for relaxation. Aim for pleasure.

Once you are settled, close your eyes or bring them to a soft gaze—whichever brings relaxation to your eyes.

Now, bring your attention to your breathing. Be a witness to it. Notice. Is it fast? Is it slow? Is it deep? Is it shallow? Witness your breathing body like you would calmly witness a new baby discovering its feet for the first time. simply be with it. Feel your inhales and exhales.

You can now become a bit more active with your breath. If you feel a desire to change your breathing at all—perhaps change its rhythm—please do. Maybe you notice you would like to take a deep breath in and let out a sigh. Maybe you feel like doing a little rapid breathing to free it up. Or maybe it's all good just how it is. simply take a moment to experiment with your breath.

Once you have made any desired changes, bring yourself back to the passive witness state again. Be with your breathing. Be with your body. Be with yourself.

Grounding the Body

Bring your attention deep into your lower abdomen, focusing simply in front of the spine at the core of your body. Imagine there is a cylindrical tube that attaches this point in your body to the surface of the Earth. You can imagine this tube to be whatever you choose: a hose, a root, a tree trunk, a lava tube, a ray of light. Really see it in your mind's eye and imagine it connecting the center of you with the Earth.

On your next exhale, imagine your tube sinking deeper into the Earth. It falls easily. It gets longer and longer. It falls through all the layers of the Earth. It falls through rock, water, and magma—all the way down to the very center of the Earth. Feel it as the core of your body firmly attaches to the core of Mother Earth. Your bottom is heavy and you feel your connection.

On your next exhale, imagine taking all the energy you don't need right now and sending it down through the tube. Give it to Mother Earth. You don't have to see it or know what it is, simply suggest to yourself that you're letting go of whatever isn't needed right now. It is falling toward the center of the Earth. Where there is tension or pain in your body, relax the area and let it all drain into Mother Earth. This is her compost; she will take it and turn it into fertile soil.

Try to match your breathing with your release: on your inhale, gather all your undesirable energy into a blob of goo and then on your exhale, let it drop down your tube into the Earth. Or you can be more physical about it. On your inhale, stand up and tense your muscles, bringing in and intensifying the energy, and then on your

exhale, release all your muscles and fall over or into your seat.

Take some time to practice this on your own for a bit, unguided. During this time, give whatever you want over to Mother Earth through your grounding cord.

Now, take a moment to stop your download and simply feel yourself, feel your grounding cord. Be with what is for a few moments. Bring your attention back to the room slowly. If your eyes are closed, open them slowly. Wiggle your body around a bit. Do what you need to do to bring your awareness back into the room and be present with the people who are here.

2. The Neutrality Exercise: Bodily Fluids

Take a moment to contemplate bodily fluids. Whatever your mind lands on related to bodily fluids, take a moment to be with it. Notice how you feel and the thoughts running through your mind being present with whatever your mind lands on as you contemplate bodily fluids. Be there, be with how you are feeling, and be with the thoughts that come to your mind. (Allow 30–60 seconds to pass.)

Next, imagine there is a sheet of glass between you and whatever your mind lands on as you contemplate bodily fluids. Notice. Do your feelings change at all when you look at bodily fluids through a sheet of glass? Do your thoughts change? Notice how you feel and the thoughts that come to your mind having a sheet of glass between you and whatever your mind lands on as you contemplate bodily fluids. (Allow 30–60 seconds to pass.)

Now, image you are in a huge room—think of a ballroom or a large conference room. Whatever your mind lands on as you contemplate bodily fluids is at one end of the room and you are at the other; you can see it, but from far away. Investigate how this feels and what thoughts arise in your mind. Did your reaction change at all from the prior scenarios? (Allow 30–60 seconds to pass.)

And now, imagine you are at the top of a tall tower, and whatever your mind lands on as you contemplate bodily fluids is outside the tower, down on the ground far below you. See what this feels like and what thoughts come to your mind. (Allow 30–60 seconds to pass.)

Finally, return to contemplating bodily fluids. Be with how you feel and the thoughts that come to your mind as you contemplate bodily fluids. (Allow 30–60 seconds to pass.)

3. Presence Yourself

Before you step away completely, take a moment to bring your awareness back into the present moment. Open your eyes and look around you. See what is in the space with you. Hear the sounds that are around you. Feel the air around you and the body you are living in. You can even pay attention to what you are tasting and smelling. Take some moments to bring your attention to the present moment and away from the topic you just explored.

4. Introspection

How was that for you?

What did you learn about yourself?

Did any of your reactions surprise you?

How will you bring the experience of working The Neutrality Exercise on this topic into your life?

Topic 7: Skin to Skin

1. A Basic Grounding

Bringing Attention to Your Breath

You can sit, stand, lie down, or do whatever works best for you. Our aim is to have your body in a state of balance, release, and maybe even in a state of pleasure. If you are seated, your weight should be evenly distributed on your sit bones. If you are standing, keep your weight evenly distributed between your feet. If you are pregnant and lying down, do so on your left side with pillows to support you. If you are not pregnant and want to lie down, do so on your back, perhaps with your knees up and feet on the ground if that is more comfortable for you. Aim for comfort. Aim for relaxation. Aim for pleasure.

Once you are settled, close your eyes or bring them to a soft gaze—whichever brings relaxation to your eyes.

Now, bring your attention to your breathing. Be a witness to it. Notice. Is it fast? Is it slow? Is it deep? Is it shallow? Witness your breathing body like you would calmly witness a new baby discovering its feet for the first time. simply be with it. Feel your inhales and exhales.

You can now become a bit more active with your breath. If you feel a desire to change your breathing at all—perhaps change its rhythm—please do. Maybe you notice you would like to take a deep breath in and let out a sigh. Maybe you feel like doing a little rapid breathing to free it up. Or maybe it's all good just how it is. simply take a moment to experiment with your breath.

Once you have made any desired changes, bring yourself back to the passive witness state again. Be with your breathing. Be with your body. Be with yourself.

Grounding the Body

Bring your attention deep into your lower abdomen, focusing simply in front of the spine at the core of your body. Imagine there is a cylindrical tube that attaches this point in your body to the surface of the Earth. You can imagine this tube to be whatever you choose: a hose, a root, a tree trunk, a lava tube, a ray of light. Really see it in your mind's eye and imagine it connecting the center of you with the Earth.

On your next exhale, imagine your tube sinking deeper into the Earth. It falls easily. It gets longer and longer. It falls through all the layers of the Earth. It falls through rock, water, and magma—all the way down to the very center of the Earth. Feel it as the core of your body firmly attaches to the core of Mother Earth. Your bottom is heavy and you feel your connection.

On your next exhale, imagine taking all the energy you don't need right now and sending it down through the tube. Give it to Mother Earth. You don't have to see it or know what it is, simply suggest to yourself that you're letting go of whatever isn't needed right now. It is falling toward the center of the Earth. Where there is tension or pain in your body, relax the area and let it all drain into Mother Earth. This is her compost; she will take it and turn it into fertile soil.

Try to match your breathing with your release: on your inhale, gather all your undesirable energy into a blob of goo and then on your exhale, let it drop down your tube into the Earth. Or you can be more physical about it. On your inhale, stand up and tense your muscles, bringing in and intensifying the energy, and then on your

exhale, release all your muscles and fall over or into your seat.

Take some time to practice this on your own for a bit, unguided. During this time, give whatever you want over to Mother Earth through your grounding cord.

Now, take a moment to stop your download and simply feel yourself, feel your grounding cord. Be with what is for a few moments. Bring your attention back to the room slowly. If your eyes are closed, open them slowly. Wiggle your body around a bit. Do what you need to do to bring your awareness back into the room and be present with the people who are here.

2. The Neutrality Exercise: Skin to Skin

Imagine you are in the presence of your client and their newborn baby. Be in their presence. Notice how you feel and the thoughts that come to your mind being there with them. Be there. Be with your thoughts and be with your feelings. (Allow 30–60 seconds to pass.)

Now, notice that your client is bare chested and their newborn has nothing on their skin whatsoever. Baby is resting nude on their parent's bare chest—skin to skin. Be in their presence. Notice how you feel and the thoughts that come to your mind being there with them. Be there. Be with your thoughts. And be with your feelings. (Allow 30–60 seconds to pass.)

Next, imagine there is a sheet of glass between you and your client and their newborn as they lay skin-to-skin. Notice. Do your feelings or thoughts change when you look at them through a sheet of glass? Notice how you feel and the thoughts that come to your mind being in a room with them while having a sheet of glass between you. (Allow 30–60 seconds to pass.)

Now, image you are in a huge room—think of a ballroom or a large conference room. Imagine your client and their newborn are resting skin-to-skin at the opposite end of the room from you; you can see them, but they are far away. Investigate how this is for you and whether your thoughts or feelings change from the prior scenarios. (Allow 30–60 seconds to pass.)

Go back to simply being in the room with your client and their newborn. Simply be in their presence. Notice how you feel and the thoughts that come to your mind being there with them. Be there. Be with your thoughts and feelings. (Allow 30–60 seconds to pass.)

Then you come to notice that your client and newborn are snuggling fully clothed. Be in their presence. Notice how you feel and the thoughts that come to your mind being there with them snuggling with all their clothes on. Be there. Be with your thoughts. And be with your feelings. (Allow 30–60 seconds to pass.)

Next, imagine there is a sheet of glass between you and your client and their newborn snuggling with their clothes on. Notice. Do your feelings or thoughts change when you look at them through a sheet of glass? Notice how you feel and the thoughts that come to your mind being in the room with them while having a sheet of glass between you and them. (Allow 30–60 seconds to pass.)

Now, image you are in a huge room. Imagine your client and their newborn are snuggling fully clothed at the opposite end of the room from you; you can see them, but from far away. Investigate how this feels. Investigate the thoughts that enter your mind watching your client and their newborn snuggle fully clothed far away from you. (Allow 30–60 seconds to pass.)

Finally, return to simply being in the room with your client and their newborn snuggling. Be there in the room with them. Notice how you are feeling. Notice your thoughts. Notice which scenario your mind lands upon. Be there, and be with your thoughts and feelings. (Allow 30–60 seconds to pass.)

3. Presence Yourself

Before you step away completely, take a moment to bring your awareness back into the present moment. Open your eyes and look around you. See what is in the space with you. Hear the sounds that are around you. Feel the air around you and the body you are living in. You can even pay attention to what you are tasting and smelling. Take some moments to bring your attention to the present moment and away from the topic you just explored.

4. Introspection

How was that for you?

What did you learn about yourself?

Did any of your reactions surprise you?

How will you bring the experience of working The Neutrality Exercise on this topic into your life?

Topic 8: Breastfeeding

1. A Basic Grounding

Bringing Attention to Your Breath

You can sit, stand, lie down, or do whatever works best for you. Our aim is to have your body in a state of balance, release, and maybe even in a state of pleasure. If you are seated, your weight should be evenly distributed on your sit bones. If you are standing, keep your weight evenly distributed between your feet. If you are pregnant and lying down, do so on your left side with pillows to support you. If you are not pregnant and want to lie down, do so on your back, perhaps with your knees up and feet on the ground if that is more comfortable for you. Aim for comfort. Aim for relaxation. Aim for pleasure.

Once you are settled, close your eyes or bring them to a soft gaze—whichever brings relaxation to your eyes.

Now, bring your attention to your breathing. Be a witness to it. Notice. Is it fast? Is it slow? Is it deep? Is it shallow? Witness your breathing body like you would calmly witness a new baby discovering its feet for the first time. simply be with it. Feel your inhales and exhales.

You can now become a bit more active with your breath. If you feel a desire to change your breathing at all—perhaps change its rhythm—please do. Maybe you notice you would like to take a deep breath in and let out a sigh. Maybe you feel like doing a little rapid breathing to free it up. Or maybe it's all good just how it is. simply take a moment to experiment with your breath.

Once you have made any desired changes, bring yourself back to the passive witness state again. Be with your breathing. Be with your body. Be with yourself.

Grounding the Body

Bring your attention deep into your lower abdomen, focusing simply in front of the spine at the core of your body. Imagine there is a cylindrical tube that attaches this point in your body to the surface of the Earth. You can imagine this tube to be whatever you choose: a hose, a root, a tree trunk, a lava tube, a ray of light. Really see it in your mind's eye and imagine it connecting the center of you with the Earth.

On your next exhale, imagine your tube sinking deeper into the Earth. It falls easily. It gets longer and longer. It falls through all the layers of the Earth. It falls through rock, water, and magma—all the way down to the very center of the Earth. Feel it as the core of your body firmly attaches to the core of Mother Earth. Your bottom is heavy and you feel your connection.

On your next exhale, imagine taking all the energy you don't need right now and sending it down through the tube. Give it to Mother Earth. You don't have to see it or know what it is, simply suggest to yourself that you're letting go of whatever isn't needed right now. It is falling toward the center of the Earth. Where there is tension or pain in your body, relax the area and let it all drain into Mother Earth. This is her compost; she will take it and turn it into fertile soil.

Try to match your breathing with your release: on your inhale, gather all your undesirable energy into a blob of goo and then on your exhale, let it drop down your tube into the Earth. Or you can be more physical about it. On your inhale, stand up and tense your muscles, bringing in and intensifying the energy, and then on your

exhale, release all your muscles and fall over or into your seat.

Take some time to practice this on your own for a bit, unguided. During this time, give whatever you want over to Mother Earth through your grounding cord.

Now, take a moment to stop your download and simply feel yourself, feel your grounding cord. Be with what is for a few moments. Bring your attention back to the room slowly. If your eyes are closed, open them slowly. Wiggle your body around a bit. Do what you need to do to bring your awareness back into the room and be present with the people who are here.

2. The Neutrality Exercise: Breastfeeding

Imagine you are in the presence of a baby while it is breastfeeding. Be there with the breastfeeding team. Notice how you feel and the thoughts that come to your mind being there with them. Be with them. Be with your thoughts and be with your feelings. (Allow 30–60 seconds to pass.)

Next, imagine there is a sheet of glass between you and the breastfeeding team. Do your feelings or thoughts change? Notice how you feel and the thoughts that come to your mind watching a baby breastfeed through a sheet of glass. (Allow 30–60 seconds to pass.)

Now, image you are in a huge room—think of a ballroom or a large conference room. You sit at one end of the room. On the opposite end of the room, you know there is a baby breastfeeding. You know they are there, but you can't see them very clearly. Notice how you feel being there. Notice the thoughts that come to your mind. Be in the room with them and be with your thoughts and feelings. (Allow

30–60 seconds to pass.)

And now, imagine you are at the top of a tall tower, and down on the ground below you is a baby breastfeeding. See what it feels like and the thoughts that come to your mind imagining this scenario. (Allow 30–60 seconds to pass.)

Finally, go back to simply being in the room with a breastfeeding baby. Be there. Notice your thoughts. Notice your feelings. (Allow 30–60 seconds to pass.)

3. Presence Yourself

Before you step away completely, take a moment to bring your awareness back into the present moment. Open your eyes and look around you. See what is in the space with you. Hear the sounds that are around you. Feel the air around you and the body you are living in. You can even pay attention to what you are tasting and smelling. Take some moments to bring your attention to the present moment and away from the topic you just explored.

4. Introspection

How was that for you?

What did you learn about yourself?

Did any of your reactions surprise you?

How will you bring the experience of working The Neutrality Exercise on this topic into your life?

Topic 9: Formula

1. A Basic Grounding

Bringing Attention to Your Breath

You can sit, stand, lie down, or do whatever works best for you. Our aim is to have your body in a state of balance, release, and maybe even in a state of pleasure. If you are seated, your weight should be evenly distributed on your sit bones. If you are standing, keep your weight evenly distributed between your feet. If you are pregnant and lying down, do so on your left side with pillows to support you. If you are not pregnant and want to lie down, do so on your back, perhaps with your knees up and feet on the ground if that is more comfortable for you. Aim for comfort. Aim for relaxation. Aim for pleasure.

Once you are settled, close your eyes or bring them to a soft gaze—whichever brings relaxation to your eyes.

Now, bring your attention to your breathing. Be a witness to it. Notice. Is it fast? Is it slow? Is it deep? Is it shallow? Witness your breathing body like you would calmly witness a new baby discovering its feet for the first time. simply be with it. Feel your inhales and exhales.

You can now become a bit more active with your breath. If you feel a desire to change your breathing at all—perhaps change its rhythm—please do. Maybe you notice you would like to take a deep breath in and let out a sigh. Maybe you feel like doing a little rapid breathing to free it up. Or maybe it's all good just how it is. simply take a moment to experiment with your breath.

Once you have made any desired changes, bring yourself back to the passive witness state again. Be with your breathing. Be with your body. Be with yourself.

Grounding the Body

Bring your attention deep into your lower abdomen, focusing simply in front of the spine at the core of your body. Imagine there is a cylindrical tube that attaches this point in your body to the surface of the Earth. You can imagine this tube to be whatever you choose: a hose, a root, a tree trunk, a lava tube, a ray of light. Really see it in your mind's eye and imagine it connecting the center of you with the Earth.

On your next exhale, imagine your tube sinking deeper into the Earth. It falls easily. It gets longer and longer. It falls through all the layers of the Earth. It falls through rock, water, and magma—all the way down to the very center of the Earth. Feel it as the core of your body firmly attaches to the core of Mother Earth. Your bottom is heavy and you feel your connection.

On your next exhale, imagine taking all the energy you don't need right now and sending it down through the tube. Give it to Mother Earth. You don't have to see it or know what it is, simply suggest to yourself that you're letting go of whatever isn't needed right now. It is falling toward the center of the Earth. Where there is tension or pain in your body, relax the area and let it all drain into Mother Earth. This is her compost; she will take it and turn it into fertile soil.

Try to match your breathing with your release: on your inhale, gather all your undesirable energy into a blob of goo and then on your exhale, let it drop down your tube into the Earth. Or you can be more physical about it. On your inhale, stand up and tense your muscles, bringing in and intensifying the energy, and then on your

exhale, release all your muscles and fall over or into your seat.

Take some time to practice this on your own for a bit, unguided. During this time, give whatever you want over to Mother Earth through your grounding cord.

Now, take a moment to stop your download and simply feel yourself, feel your grounding cord. Be with what is for a few moments. Bring your attention back to the room slowly. If your eyes are closed, open them slowly. Wiggle your body around a bit. Do what you need to do to bring your awareness back into the room and be present with the people who are here.

2. The Neutrality Exercise: Formula

Imagine you are in the presence of a baby being formula fed. Be in their presence. Notice how you feel being there with them. Be there, and be with your thoughts and feelings. (Allow 30–60 seconds to pass.)

Next, imagine there is a sheet of glass between you and the baby being formula fed. Notice. Do your feelings change when you look at them through a sheet of glass? Notice what it is like for you to watch through a sheet of glass as a baby is being formula fed. Notice your thoughts and feelings. (Allow 30–60 seconds to pass.)

Now, image you are in a huge room—think of a ballroom or large conference room. Imagine that you are at one end of the room and on the opposite end of the room there is a baby being formula fed. You can see them, but they are far away. Notice how this is for you and whether your feelings or thoughts change from the prior scenarios. (Allow 30–60 seconds to pass.)

And now, imagine you are at the top of a tall tower, and down on the ground below you is a baby being formula fed. See what it feels like and what thoughts arise in your mind as you imagine a scenario where you are at the top of a tall tower looking down below at a baby being formula fed. Notice the feelings and thoughts that arise as you imagine. (Allow 30–60 seconds to pass.)

Finally, return to simply being with a baby being formula fed. Be there with them. Notice your thoughts. Notice your feelings. Be with it all. (Allow 30–60 seconds to pass.)

3. Presence Yourself

Before you step away completely, take a moment to bring your awareness back into the present moment. Open your eyes and look around you. See what is in the space with you. Hear the sounds that are around you. Feel the air around you and the body you are living in. You can even pay attention to what you are tasting and smelling. Take some moments to bring your attention to the present moment and away from the topic you just explored.

4. Introspection

How was that for you?

What did you learn about yourself?

Did any of your reactions surprise you?

How will you bring the experience of working The Neutrality Exercise on this topic into your life?

Topic 10: Midwife

1. A Basic Grounding

Bringing Attention to Your Breath

You can sit, stand, lie down, or do whatever works best for you. Our aim is to have your body in a state of balance, release, and maybe even in a state of pleasure. If you are seated, your weight should be evenly distributed on your sit bones. If you are standing, keep your weight evenly distributed between your feet. If you are pregnant and lying down, do so on your left side with pillows to support you. If you are not pregnant and want to lie down, do so on your back, perhaps with your knees up and feet on the ground if that is more comfortable for you. Aim for comfort. Aim for relaxation. Aim for pleasure.

Once you are settled, close your eyes or bring them to a soft gaze—whichever brings relaxation to your eyes.

Now, bring your attention to your breathing. Be a witness to it. Notice. Is it fast? Is it slow? Is it deep? Is it shallow? Witness your breathing body like you would calmly witness a new baby discovering its feet for the first time. simply be with it. Feel your inhales and exhales.

You can now become a bit more active with your breath. If you feel a desire to change your breathing at all—perhaps change its rhythm—please do. Maybe you notice you would like to take a deep breath in and let out a sigh. Maybe you feel like doing a little rapid breathing to free it up. Or maybe it's all good just how it is. simply take a moment to experiment with your breath.

Once you have made any desired changes, bring yourself back to the passive witness state again. Be with your breathing. Be with your body. Be with yourself.

Grounding the Body

Bring your attention deep into your lower abdomen, focusing simply in front of the spine at the core of your body. Imagine there is a cylindrical tube that attaches this point in your body to the surface of the Earth. You can imagine this tube to be whatever you choose: a hose, a root, a tree trunk, a lava tube, a ray of light. Really see it in your mind's eye and imagine it connecting the center of you with the Earth.

On your next exhale, imagine your tube sinking deeper into the Earth. It falls easily. It gets longer and longer. It falls through all the layers of the Earth. It falls through rock, water, and magma—all the way down to the very center of the Earth. Feel it as the core of your body firmly attaches to the core of Mother Earth. Your bottom is heavy and you feel your connection.

On your next exhale, imagine taking all the energy you don't need right now and sending it down through the tube. Give it to Mother Earth. You don't have to see it or know what it is, simply suggest to yourself that you're letting go of whatever isn't needed right now. It is falling toward the center of the Earth. Where there is tension or pain in your body, relax the area and let it all drain into Mother Earth. This is her compost; she will take it and turn it into fertile soil.

Try to match your breathing with your release: on your inhale, gather all your undesirable energy into a blob of goo and then on your exhale, let it drop down your tube into the Earth. Or you can be more physical about it. On your inhale, stand up and tense your muscles, bringing in and intensifying the energy, and then on your

exhale, release all your muscles and fall over or into your seat.

Take some time to practice this on your own for a bit, unguided. During this time, give whatever you want over to Mother Earth through your grounding cord.

Now, take a moment to stop your download and simply feel yourself, feel your grounding cord. Be with what is for a few moments. Bring your attention back to the room slowly. If your eyes are closed, open them slowly. Wiggle your body around a bit. Do what you need to do to bring your awareness back into the room and be present with the people who are here.

2. The Neutrality Exercise: Midwife

Take a moment to contemplate pregnancy. Really imagine what that word means to you: pregnancy. Notice how you feel and the thoughts that run through your mind as you contemplate pregnancy. Be there, be with how you are feeling, and be with the thoughts that arise in your mind. (Allow 30–60 seconds to pass.)

Next, imagine there is a sheet of glass between you and whatever your mind lands on as you contemplate pregnancy. Notice. Do your feelings change at all while you look through a sheet of glass at whatever comes to your mind as you contemplate pregnancy? Do your thoughts change? Notice how you feel and the thoughts that come to your mind having a sheet of glass between you and whatever your mind lands on as you contemplate pregnancy. (Allow 30–60 seconds to pass.)

Now, image you are in a huge room—think of a ballroom or a large conference room. Whatever your mind lands on as you contemplate pregnancy is at one end of the room and you are at the other.

Investigate how this feels and what thoughts arise in your mind as you look at whatever comes to your mind as you contemplate pregnancy on the opposite end of a large room from you. Did your reaction change at all from the prior scenarios? (Allow 30–60 seconds to pass.)

And now, imagine you are at the top of a tall tower, and whatever your mind lands on as you contemplate pregnancy is outside the tower, down on the ground far below you. See what this feels like and notice the thoughts that come to your mind as you look far below you at whatever comes to your mind as you contemplate pregnancy. (Allow 30–60 seconds to pass.)

Finally, return to simply being with the word pregnancy again. Be with how you feel and the thoughts that come to your mind. (Allow 30–60 seconds to pass.)

3. Presence Yourself

Before you step away completely, take a moment to bring your awareness back into the present moment. Open your eyes and look around you. See what is in the space with you. Hear the sounds that are around you. Feel the air around you and the body you are living in. You can even pay attention to what you are tasting and smelling. Take some moments to bring your attention to the present moment and away from the topic you just explored.

4. Introspection

How was that for you?

What did you learn about yourself?

Did any of your reactions surprise you?

How will you bring the experience of working The Neutrality Exercise on this topic into your life?

Topic 11: Obstetrician (OB)

1. A Basic Grounding

Bringing Attention to Your Breath

You can sit, stand, lie down, or do whatever works best for you. Our aim is to have your body in a state of balance, release, and maybe even in a state of pleasure. If you are seated, your weight should be evenly distributed on your sit bones. If you are standing, keep your weight evenly distributed between your feet. If you are pregnant and lying down, do so on your left side with pillows to support you. If you are not pregnant and want to lie down, do so on your back, perhaps with your knees up and feet on the ground if that is more comfortable for you. Aim for comfort. Aim for relaxation. Aim for pleasure.

Once you are settled, close your eyes or bring them to a soft gaze—whichever brings relaxation to your eyes.

Now, bring your attention to your breathing. Be a witness to it. Notice. Is it fast? Is it slow? Is it deep? Is it shallow? Witness your breathing body like you would calmly witness a new baby discovering its feet for the first time. simply be with it. Feel your inhales and exhales.

You can now become a bit more active with your breath. If you feel a desire to change your breathing at all—perhaps change its rhythm—please do. Maybe you notice you would like to take a deep breath in and let out a sigh. Maybe you feel like doing a little rapid breathing to free it up. Or maybe it's all good just how it is. simply take a moment to experiment with your breath.

Once you have made any desired changes, bring yourself back to the passive witness state again. Be with your breathing. Be with your body. Be with yourself.

Grounding the Body

Bring your attention deep into your lower abdomen, focusing simply in front of the spine at the core of your body. Imagine there is a cylindrical tube that attaches this point in your body to the surface of the Earth. You can imagine this tube to be whatever you choose: a hose, a root, a tree trunk, a lava tube, a ray of light. Really see it in your mind's eye and imagine it connecting the center of you with the Earth.

On your next exhale, imagine your tube sinking deeper into the Earth. It falls easily. It gets longer and longer. It falls through all the layers of the Earth. It falls through rock, water, and magma—all the way down to the very center of the Earth. Feel it as the core of your body firmly attaches to the core of Mother Earth. Your bottom is heavy and you feel your connection.

On your next exhale, imagine taking all the energy you don't need right now and sending it down through the tube. Give it to Mother Earth. You don't have to see it or know what it is, simply suggest to yourself that you're letting go of whatever isn't needed right now. It is falling toward the center of the Earth. Where there is tension or pain in your body, relax the area and let it all drain into Mother Earth. This is her compost; she will take it and turn it into fertile soil.

Try to match your breathing with your release: on your inhale, gather all your undesirable energy into a blob of goo and then on your exhale, let it drop down your tube into the Earth. Or you can be more physical about it. On your inhale, stand up and tense your muscles, bringing in and intensifying the energy, and then on your

84

exhale, release all your muscles and fall over or into your seat.

Take some time to practice this on your own for a bit, unguided. During this time, give whatever you want over to Mother Earth through your grounding cord.

Now, take a moment to stop your download and simply feel yourself, feel your grounding cord. Be with what is for a few moments. Bring your attention back to the room slowly. If your eyes are closed, open them slowly. Wiggle your body around a bit. Do what you need to do to bring your awareness back into the room and be present with the people who are here.

2. The Neutrality Exercise: Obstetrician (OB)

Imagine you are in the presence of an obstetrician (OB). Be in their presence. Notice how you feel and the thoughts that come into your mind being there with an OB. Be there. Be with your thoughts. And be with your feelings. (Allow 30–60 seconds to pass.)

Next, imagine there is a sheet of glass between you and an OB. Notice. Do your feelings or thoughts change when you look at them through a sheet of glass? Notice how you feel and the thoughts that come to your mind being with an OB when there is a sheet of glass between you. (Allow 30–60 seconds to pass.)

Now, image you are in a huge room—think of a ballroom or a large conference room. An OB is at the opposite end of the room from you. You can see them, but they are far away. Investigate how this feels. Investigate your thoughts. Notice whether your thoughts or feelings change from the prior scenarios. (Allow 30–60 seconds to pass.)

And now, imagine you are at the top of a tall tower, and an OB is down on the ground far below you. Do your thoughts change? Do your feelings change? Be with your thoughts and feelings as you ponder this scenario. (Allow 30–60 seconds to pass.)

Finally, return to simply being present with an OB. Be there in with them and notice how it is for you. Be there. Be with your thoughts and be with your feelings. (Allow 30–60 seconds to pass.)

3. Presence Yourself

Before you step away completely, take a moment to bring your awareness back into the present moment. Open your eyes and look around you. See what is in the space with you. Hear the sounds that are around you. Feel the air around you and the body you are living in. You can even pay attention to what you are tasting and smelling. Take some moments to bring your attention to the present moment and away from the topic you just explored.

4. Introspection

How was that for you?

What did you learn about yourself?

Did any of your reactions surprise you?

How will you bring the experience of working The Neutrality Exercise on this topic into your life?

Topic 12: Provider

1. A Basic Grounding

Bringing Attention to Your Breath

You can sit, stand, lie down, or do whatever works best for you. Our aim is to have your body in a state of balance, release, and maybe even in a state of pleasure. If you are seated, your weight should be evenly distributed on your sit bones. If you are standing, keep your weight evenly distributed between your feet. If you are pregnant and lying down, do so on your left side with pillows to support you. If you are not pregnant and want to lie down, do so on your back, perhaps with your knees up and feet on the ground if that is more comfortable for you. Aim for comfort. Aim for relaxation. Aim for pleasure.

Once you are settled, close your eyes or bring them to a soft gaze—whichever brings relaxation to your eyes.

Now, bring your attention to your breathing. Be a witness to it. Notice. Is it fast? Is it slow? Is it deep? Is it shallow? Witness your breathing body like you would calmly witness a new baby discovering its feet for the first time. simply be with it. Feel your inhales and exhales.

You can now become a bit more active with your breath. If you feel a desire to change your breathing at all—perhaps change its rhythm—please do. Maybe you notice you would like to take a deep breath in and let out a sigh. Maybe you feel like doing a little rapid breathing to free it up. Or maybe it's all good just how it is. simply take a moment to experiment with your breath.

Once you have made any desired changes, bring yourself back to the passive witness state again. Be with your breathing. Be with your body. Be with yourself.

Grounding the Body

Bring your attention deep into your lower abdomen, focusing simply in front of the spine at the core of your body. Imagine there is a cylindrical tube that attaches this point in your body to the surface of the Earth. You can imagine this tube to be whatever you choose: a hose, a root, a tree trunk, a lava tube, a ray of light. Really see it in your mind's eye and imagine it connecting the center of you with the Earth.

On your next exhale, imagine your tube sinking deeper into the Earth. It falls easily. It gets longer and longer. It falls through all the layers of the Earth. It falls through rock, water, and magma—all the way down to the very center of the Earth. Feel it as the core of your body firmly attaches to the core of Mother Earth. Your bottom is heavy and you feel your connection.

On your next exhale, imagine taking all the energy you don't need right now and sending it down through the tube. Give it to Mother Earth. You don't have to see it or know what it is, simply suggest to yourself that you're letting go of whatever isn't needed right now. It is falling toward the center of the Earth. Where there is tension or pain in your body, relax the area and let it all drain into Mother Earth. This is her compost; she will take it and turn it into fertile soil.

Try to match your breathing with your release: on your inhale, gather all your undesirable energy into a blob of goo and then on your exhale, let it drop down your tube into the Earth. Or you can be more physical about it. On your inhale, stand up and tense your muscles, bringing in and intensifying the energy, and then on your

90

exhale, release all your muscles and fall over or into your seat.

Take some time to practice this on your own for a bit, unguided. During this time, give whatever you want over to Mother Earth through your grounding cord.

Now, take a moment to stop your download and simply feel yourself, feel your grounding cord. Be with what is for a few moments. Bring your attention back to the room slowly. If your eyes are closed, open them slowly. Wiggle your body around a bit. Do what you need to do to bring your awareness back into the room and be present with the people who are here.

2. The Neutrality Exercise: Provider

Imagine your client is in labor and the provider your client chose to attend the birth of their baby is there with you. Be in their presence. Notice how you feel and the thoughts that come to your mind being there with them. Be there with them, and be with your thoughts and feelings. (Allow 30–60 seconds to pass.)

Now, notice that their provider is starting to do things to your laboring client that you don't agree with. Be with how you feel and the thoughts that come to your mind imagining their provider doing things to your laboring client that you do not agree with. Be there, and be with your thoughts and feelings. (Allow 30–60 seconds to pass.)

Next, imagine there is a sheet of glass between you and your laboring client as their provider does things to your client that you do not agree with. Notice. Do your feelings or thoughts change when you look at them through a sheet of glass? Notice how you feel and the thoughts that come to your mind watching this through a sheet of glass. (Allow 30–60 seconds to pass.)

Now, image you are in a huge room—think of a ballroom or a large conference room. Imagine you are at one end of the room and on the other end of the room your client's provider is doing things to them that you do not agree with. You can see them, but they are far away. Investigate how this feels. Investigate the thoughts that arise in your mind. Notice whether anything changes for you compared to the prior scenarios. (Allow 30–60 seconds to pass.)

Go back to simply being in the room with your laboring client and their provider. Be in their presence. Notice how you feel and the thoughts that come to your mind being there with them. Be there. Be with your thoughts. And be with your feelings. (Allow 30–60 seconds to pass.)

Now, come to notice that their provider is doing every single thing exactly the way you think they should be doing it. Be in their presence. Notice how you feel and the thoughts that come to your mind being there with them as they do everything exactly the way you think they should be done. Be there, and be with your thoughts and feelings. (Allow 30–60 seconds to pass.)

Next, imagine there is a sheet of glass between you and your client as their provider does every single thing exactly the way you think they should be done. Notice. Do your feelings change when you look at them through a sheet of glass? Notice how you feel being in the room with them while having a sheet of glass between you. Be with your thoughts and be with your feelings. (Allow 30–60 seconds to pass.)

Now, image you are in a huge room. Imagine you are at one end of the room and on the other end of the room is your client and their provider doing things exactly how you think they should be done.

You can barely see them, but you know they are there. Investigate how this feels. Investigate the thoughts that arise in your mind. Has anything changed within you since pondering the prior scenarios? (Allow 30–60 seconds to pass.)

Finally, return to simply being in the room with your laboring client and their provider. Be there in the room with them; notice how you are feeling and the thoughts that come to your mind. Also notice which scenario your mind comes to rest upon. (Allow 30–60 seconds to pass.)

3. Presence Yourself

Before you step away completely, take a moment to bring your awareness back into the present moment. Open your eyes and look around you. See what is in the space with you. Hear the sounds that are around you. Feel the air around you and the body you are living in. You can even pay attention to what you are tasting and smelling. Take some moments to bring your attention to the present moment and away from the topic you simply explored.

4. Introspection

How was that for you?

What did you learn about yourself?

Did any of your reactions surprise you?

How will you bring the experience of working The Neutrality Exercise on this topic into your life?

Topic 13: Monitoring

1. A Basic Grounding

Bringing Attention to Your Breath

You can sit, stand, lie down, or do whatever works best for you. Our aim is to have your body in a state of balance, release, and maybe even in a state of pleasure. If you are seated, your weight should be evenly distributed on your sit bones. If you are standing, keep your weight evenly distributed between your feet. If you are pregnant and lying down, do so on your left side with pillows to support you. If you are not pregnant and want to lie down, do so on your back, perhaps with your knees up and feet on the ground if that is more comfortable for you. Aim for comfort. Aim for relaxation. Aim for pleasure.

Once you are settled, close your eyes or bring them to a soft gaze—whichever brings relaxation to your eyes.

Now, bring your attention to your breathing. Be a witness to it. Notice. Is it fast? Is it slow? Is it deep? Is it shallow? Witness your breathing body like you would calmly witness a new baby discovering its feet for the first time. simply be with it. Feel your inhales and exhales.

You can now become a bit more active with your breath. If you feel a desire to change your breathing at all—perhaps change its rhythm—please do. Maybe you notice you would like to take a deep breath in and let out a sigh. Maybe you feel like doing a little rapid breathing to free it up. Or maybe it's all good just how it is. simply take a moment to experiment with your breath.

Once you have made any desired changes, bring yourself back to the passive witness state again. Be with your breathing. Be with your body. Be with yourself.

Grounding the Body

Bring your attention deep into your lower abdomen, focusing simply in front of the spine at the core of your body. Imagine there is a cylindrical tube that attaches this point in your body to the surface of the Earth. You can imagine this tube to be whatever you choose: a hose, a root, a tree trunk, a lava tube, a ray of light. Really see it in your mind's eye and imagine it connecting the center of you with the Earth.

On your next exhale, imagine your tube sinking deeper into the Earth. It falls easily. It gets longer and longer. It falls through all the layers of the Earth. It falls through rock, water, and magma—all the way down to the very center of the Earth. Feel it as the core of your body firmly attaches to the core of Mother Earth. Your bottom is heavy and you feel your connection.

On your next exhale, imagine taking all the energy you don't need right now and sending it down through the tube. Give it to Mother Earth. You don't have to see it or know what it is, simply suggest to yourself that you're letting go of whatever isn't needed right now. It is falling toward the center of the Earth. Where there is tension or pain in your body, relax the area and let it all drain into Mother Earth. This is her compost; she will take it and turn it into fertile soil.

Try to match your breathing with your release: on your inhale, gather all your undesirable energy into a blob of goo and then on your exhale, let it drop down your tube into the Earth. Or you can be more physical about it. On your inhale, stand up and tense your muscles, bringing in and intensifying the energy, and then on your

exhale, release all your muscles and fall over or into your seat.

Take some time to practice this on your own for a bit, unguided. During this time, give whatever you want over to Mother Earth through your grounding cord.

Now, take a moment to stop your download and simply feel yourself, feel your grounding cord. Be with what is for a few moments. Bring your attention back to the room slowly. If your eyes are closed, open them slowly. Wiggle your body around a bit. Do what you need to do to bring your awareness back into the room and be present with the people who are here.

2. The Neutrality Exercise: Monitoring

Imagine you are in the presence of your client in labor. Be in their presence. Notice how you feel and the thoughts that come to your mind being there with them. Be there. Be with your thoughts. And be with your feelings. (Allow 30–60 seconds to pass.)

Now, notice that some hours have gone by and no one has come to monitor the fetus. Be there with your client in labor knowing that no one has come to monitor the fetus in a number of hours. Imagine this scenario and be with whatever feelings or thoughts may arise in your mind. (Allow 30–60 seconds to pass.)

Next, imagine you are in a huge room — think of a ballroom or a large conference room. Imagine that you have been witnessing your laboring client for hours from across a huge room, and no one has come to monitor the fetus. Be with your feelings and thoughts as you imagine this scenario. (Allow 30–60 seconds to pass.)

Go back to simply being present with your client in labor. Be there with them, be with how you are feeling, and be with any thoughts that may arise. (Allow 30–60 seconds to pass.)

This time, you notice that your client in labor is hooked up to a continuous fetal monitor. Again, be there with them. Notice your feelings and thoughts as you witness them laboring while attached to a continuous fetal monitor. (Allow 30–60 seconds to pass.)

Next, imagine you are in a huge room. Imagine that you are witnessing your client in labor while connected to a continuous fetal monitor, far away on the other side of the room from you. Be with your feelings and thoughts as you imagine this scenario. (Allow 30–60 seconds to pass.)

Go back to simply being present with your client in labor. Be there with them, be with how you are feeling, and be with any thoughts that may arise in your mind. (Allow 30–60 seconds to pass.)

Now, notice that an hour has gone by and someone has come to monitor the fetus for some moments. Imagine this scenario where you have been with your client in labor for an hour and someone comes to monitor the fetus for some moments and leaves. Imagine this scenario and be with whatever feelings or thoughts may arise. (Allow 30–60 seconds to pass.)

Next, imagine you are in a huge room. Imagine that you have been witnessing this labor for an hour from across this huge room and someone comes to monitor the fetus for some moments. Be with your feelings and thoughts as you imagine this scenario. (Allow 30–60 seconds to pass.)

Finally, go back to simply being present with someone in labor. Imagine being in their presence. Notice how you feel and the thoughts that come to your mind being there with them. Also, notice which scenario your mind comes to rest upon: no monitoring, continuous monitoring, or intermittent monitoring. Be there, and be with your thoughts and feelings. (Allow 30–60 seconds to pass.)

3. Presence Yourself

Before you step away completely, take a moment to bring your awareness back into the present moment. Open your eyes and look around you. See what is in the space with you. Hear the sounds that are around you. Feel the air around you and the body you are living in. You can even pay attention to what you are tasting and smelling. Take some moments to bring your attention to the present moment and away from the topic you just explored.

4. Introspection

How was that for you?

What did you learn about yourself?

Did any of your reactions surprise you?

How will you bring the experience of working The Neutrality Exercise on this topic into your life?

Topic 14: Medical Procedures

1. A Basic Grounding

Bringing Attention to Your Breath

You can sit, stand, lie down, or do whatever works best for you. Our aim is to have your body in a state of balance, release, and maybe even in a state of pleasure. If you are seated, your weight should be evenly distributed on your sit bones. If you are standing, keep your weight evenly distributed between your feet. If you are pregnant and lying down, do so on your left side with pillows to support you. If you are not pregnant and want to lie down, do so on your back, perhaps with your knees up and feet on the ground if that is more comfortable for you. Aim for comfort. Aim for relaxation. Aim for pleasure.

Once you are settled, close your eyes or bring them to a soft gaze—whichever brings relaxation to your eyes.

Now, bring your attention to your breathing. Be a witness to it. Notice. Is it fast? Is it slow? Is it deep? Is it shallow? Witness your breathing body like you would calmly witness a new baby discovering its feet for the first time. simply be with it. Feel your inhales and exhales.

You can now become a bit more active with your breath. If you feel a desire to change your breathing at all—perhaps change its rhythm—please do. Maybe you notice you would like to take a deep breath in and let out a sigh. Maybe you feel like doing a little rapid breathing to free it up. Or maybe it's all good just how it is. simply take a moment to experiment with your breath.

Once you have made any desired changes, bring yourself back to the passive witness state again. Be with your breathing. Be with your body. Be with yourself.

Grounding the Body

Bring your attention deep into your lower abdomen, focusing simply in front of the spine at the core of your body. Imagine there is a cylindrical tube that attaches this point in your body to the surface of the Earth. You can imagine this tube to be whatever you choose: a hose, a root, a tree trunk, a lava tube, a ray of light. Really see it in your mind's eye and imagine it connecting the center of you with the Earth.

On your next exhale, imagine your tube sinking deeper into the Earth. It falls easily. It gets longer and longer. It falls through all the layers of the Earth. It falls through rock, water, and magma—all the way down to the very center of the Earth. Feel it as the core of your body firmly attaches to the core of Mother Earth. Your bottom is heavy and you feel your connection.

On your next exhale, imagine taking all the energy you don't need right now and sending it down through the tube. Give it to Mother Earth. You don't have to see it or know what it is, simply suggest to yourself that you're letting go of whatever isn't needed right now. It is falling toward the center of the Earth. Where there is tension or pain in your body, relax the area and let it all drain into Mother Earth. This is her compost; she will take it and turn it into fertile soil.

Try to match your breathing with your release: on your inhale, gather all your undesirable energy into a blob of goo and then on your exhale, let it drop down your tube into the Earth. Or you can be more physical about it. On your inhale, stand up and tense your muscles, bringing in and intensifying the energy, and then on your

exhale, release all your muscles and fall over or into your seat.

Take some time to practice this on your own for a bit, unguided. During this time, give whatever you want over to Mother Earth through your grounding cord.

Now, take a moment to stop your download and simply feel yourself, feel your grounding cord. Be with what is for a few moments. Bring your attention back to the room slowly. If your eyes are closed, open them slowly. Wiggle your body around a bit. Do what you need to do to bring your awareness back into the room and be present with the people who are here.

2. The Neutrality Exercise: Medical Procedures

Take a moment and contemplate the possibility of your client undergoing a medical procedure. This medical procedure could be anything you choose to place your attention upon. Pick one to run this exercise with. Pick another and do it again. Give yourself the opportunity to contemplate whatever you need to help you show up for your client. Now that you have picked a medical procedure, bring your attention to it. Notice how you feel and the thoughts running through your mind as you contemplate your client undergoing this medical procedure. (Allow 30–60 seconds to pass.)

Next, imagine there is a sheet of glass between you and your client undergoing this medical procedure. Notice. Do your feelings change at all while you look at them through a sheet of glass? Do your thoughts change? Notice how you feel and the thoughts that come to your mind while having a sheet of glass between you and your client undergoing this medical procedure. (Allow 30–60 seconds to pass.)

Now, imagine you are in a huge room—think of a ballroom or a large conference room. Imagine you are at one end of the room and your client undergoing this medical procedure is at the opposite end of the room. Investigate how this feels and whether your feelings or thoughts change from the prior scenarios. (Allow 30–60 seconds to pass.)

And now, imagine you are at the top of a tall tower, and your client undergoing this medical procedure is outside the tower, down on the ground. You can barely see them, but you know they are there. See what this feels like and witness the thoughts that come to your mind. (Allow 30–60 seconds to pass.)

Finally, return to simply being with your client undergoing this medical procedure. Be with how you feel and the thoughts that come to your mind being with your client undergoing this medical procedure. (Allow 30–60 seconds to pass.)

3. Presence Yourself

Before you step away completely, take a moment to bring your awareness back into the present moment. Open your eyes and look around you. See what is in the space with you. Hear the sounds that are around you. Feel the air around you and the body you are living in. You can even pay attention to what you are tasting and smelling. Take some moments to bring your attention to the present moment and away from the topic you just explored.

4. Introspection

How was that for you?

What did you learn about yourself?

Did any of your reactions surprise you?

How will you bring the experience of working The Neutrality Exercise on this topic into your life?

Topic 15: Schedule a Caesarean

1. A Basic Grounding

Bringing Attention to Your Breath

You can sit, stand, lie down, or do whatever works best for you. Our aim is to have your body in a state of balance, release, and maybe even in a state of pleasure. If you are seated, your weight should be evenly distributed on your sit bones. If you are standing, keep your weight evenly distributed between your feet. If you are pregnant and lying down, do so on your left side with pillows to support you. If you are not pregnant and want to lie down, do so on your back, perhaps with your knees up and feet on the ground if that is more comfortable for you. Aim for comfort. Aim for relaxation. Aim for pleasure.

Once you are settled, close your eyes or bring them to a soft gaze—whichever brings relaxation to your eyes.

Now, bring your attention to your breathing. Be a witness to it. Notice. Is it fast? Is it slow? Is it deep? Is it shallow? Witness your breathing body like you would calmly witness a new baby discovering its feet for the first time. simply be with it. Feel your inhales and exhales.

You can now become a bit more active with your breath. If you feel a desire to change your breathing at all—perhaps change its rhythm—please do. Maybe you notice you would like to take a deep breath in and let out a sigh. Maybe you feel like doing a little rapid breathing to free it up. Or maybe it's all good just how it is. simply take a moment to experiment with your breath.

Once you have made any desired changes, bring yourself back to the passive witness state again. Be with your breathing. Be with your body. Be with yourself.

Grounding the Body

Bring your attention deep into your lower abdomen, focusing simply in front of the spine at the core of your body. Imagine there is a cylindrical tube that attaches this point in your body to the surface of the Earth. You can imagine this tube to be whatever you choose: a hose, a root, a tree trunk, a lava tube, a ray of light. Really see it in your mind's eye and imagine it connecting the center of you with the Earth.

On your next exhale, imagine your tube sinking deeper into the Earth. It falls easily. It gets longer and longer. It falls through all the layers of the Earth. It falls through rock, water, and magma—all the way down to the very center of the Earth. Feel it as the core of your body firmly attaches to the core of Mother Earth. Your bottom is heavy and you feel your connection.

On your next exhale, imagine taking all the energy you don't need right now and sending it down through the tube. Give it to Mother Earth. You don't have to see it or know what it is, simply suggest to yourself that you're letting go of whatever isn't needed right now. It is falling toward the center of the Earth. Where there is tension or pain in your body, relax the area and let it all drain into Mother Earth. This is her compost; she will take it and turn it into fertile soil.

Try to match your breathing with your release: on your inhale, gather all your undesirable energy into a blob of goo and then on your exhale, let it drop down your tube into the Earth. Or you can be more physical about it. On your inhale, stand up and tense your muscles, bringing in and intensifying the energy, and then on your

exhale, release all your muscles and fall over or into your seat.

Take some time to practice this on your own for a bit, unguided. During this time, give whatever you want over to Mother Earth through your grounding cord.

Now, take a moment to stop your download and simply feel yourself, feel your grounding cord. Be with what is for a few moments. Bring your attention back to the room slowly. If your eyes are closed, open them slowly. Wiggle your body around a bit. Do what you need to do to bring your awareness back into the room and be present with the people who are here.

2. The Neutrality Exercise: Scheduled a Caesarean

Imagine you are with your pregnant client. Be in their presence. Notice how you feel and the thoughts that come to your mind being there with them. Be there. Be with your thoughts. And be with your feelings. (Allow 30–60 seconds to pass.)

Notice that their provider is suggesting that they schedule a caesarean. Notice how this is for you. Take some moments to imagine being with your client as their provider suggests that they schedule a caesarean. Be with them. And be with your thoughts and feelings. (Allow 30–60 seconds to pass.)

Next, imagine there is a sheet of glass between you and your client as their provider suggests that they schedule a caesarean. Notice. Do your thoughts or feelings change when you watch them through a sheet of glass? Notice how it is for you to watch through a sheet of glass as a provider suggests to your client that they schedule a caesarean. (Allow 30–60 seconds to pass.)

Now, image you are in a huge room—think of a ballroom or a large conference room. At one end of this room is your client whose provider is suggesting that they schedule a caesarean. You are on the opposite end of the room. You can see them, but they are far away. Investigate how this feels and what thoughts come to your mind. Does anything change for you from the prior scenarios? (Allow 30–60 seconds to pass.)

And now, imagine you are at the top of a tall tower, and down on the ground below you is your client whose provider is suggesting that they schedule a caesarean. From the top of the tower, see them far below. Witness your thoughts and feelings. Are they different than during the prior scenarios? (Allow 30–60 seconds to pass.)

Finally, return to simply being with your client. Be with them. Notice how you are feeling and what thoughts arise in your mind. (Allow 30–60 seconds to pass.)

3. Presence Yourself

Before you step away completely, take a moment to bring your awareness back into the present moment. Open your eyes and look around you. See what is in the space with you. Hear the sounds that are around you. Feel the air around you and the body you are living in. You can even pay attention to what you are tasting and smelling. Take some moments to bring your attention to the present moment and away from the topic you just explored.

4. Introspection

How was that for you?

What did you learn about yourself?

Did any of your reactions surprise you?

How will you bring the experience of working The Neutrality Exercise on this topic into your life?

Topic 16: Circumcision

1. A Basic Grounding

Bringing Attention to Your Breath

You can sit, stand, lie down, or do whatever works best for you. Our aim is to have your body in a state of balance, release, and maybe even in a state of pleasure. If you are seated, your weight should be evenly distributed on your sit bones. If you are standing, keep your weight evenly distributed between your feet. If you are pregnant and lying down, do so on your left side with pillows to support you. If you are not pregnant and want to lie down, do so on your back, perhaps with your knees up and feet on the ground if that is more comfortable for you. Aim for comfort. Aim for relaxation. Aim for pleasure.

Once you are settled, close your eyes or bring them to a soft gaze— whichever brings relaxation to your eyes.

Now, bring your attention to your breathing. Be a witness to it. Notice. Is it fast? Is it slow? Is it deep? Is it shallow? Witness your breathing body like you would calmly witness a new baby discovering its feet for the first time. simply be with it. Feel your inhales and exhales.

You can now become a bit more active with your breath. If you feel a desire to change your breathing at all—perhaps change its rhythm— please do. Maybe you notice you would like to take a deep breath in and let out a sigh. Maybe you feel like doing a little rapid breathing to free it up. Or maybe it's all good just how it is. simply take a moment to experiment with your breath.

Once you have made any desired changes, bring yourself back to the passive witness state again. Be with your breathing. Be with your body. Be with yourself.

Grounding the Body

Bring your attention deep into your lower abdomen, focusing simply in front of the spine at the core of your body. Imagine there is a cylindrical tube that attaches this point in your body to the surface of the Earth. You can imagine this tube to be whatever you choose: a hose, a root, a tree trunk, a lava tube, a ray of light. Really see it in your mind's eye and imagine it connecting the center of you with the Earth.

On your next exhale, imagine your tube sinking deeper into the Earth. It falls easily. It gets longer and longer. It falls through all the layers of the Earth. It falls through rock, water, and magma—all the way down to the very center of the Earth. Feel it as the core of your body firmly attaches to the core of Mother Earth. Your bottom is heavy and you feel your connection.

On your next exhale, imagine taking all the energy you don't need right now and sending it down through the tube. Give it to Mother Earth. You don't have to see it or know what it is, simply suggest to yourself that you're letting go of whatever isn't needed right now. It is falling toward the center of the Earth. Where there is tension or pain in your body, relax the area and let it all drain into Mother Earth. This is her compost; she will take it and turn it into fertile soil.

Try to match your breathing with your release: on your inhale, gather all your undesirable energy into a blob of goo and then on your exhale, let it drop down your tube into the Earth. Or you can be more physical about it. On your inhale, stand up and tense your muscles, bringing in and intensifying the energy, and then on your

exhale, release all your muscles and fall over or into your seat.

Take some time to practice this on your own for a bit, unguided. During this time, give whatever you want over to Mother Earth through your grounding cord.

Now, take a moment to stop your download and simply feel yourself, feel your grounding cord. Be with what is for a few moments. Bring your attention back to the room slowly. If your eyes are closed, open them slowly. Wiggle your body around a bit. Do what you need to do to bring your awareness back into the room and be present with the people who are here.

2. The Neutrality Exercise: Circumcision

Imagine you are sitting with your client. Be with them. Notice how you feel and the thoughts that come to your mind being there with them. Be there. Be with your thoughts and be with your feelings. (Allow 30–60 seconds to pass.)

Now, notice that a conversation begins on the topic of circumcision. Your client is trying to decide whether or not to circumcise their baby. Simply be present to this imagined scenario. Notice how you feel and the thoughts that arise in your mind being there with your client as they discuss the prospect of circumcising their baby. (Allow 30–60 seconds to pass.)

Next, imagine there is a sheet of glass between you and your client as they discuss whether or not to circumcise their baby. Notice. Do your feelings or thoughts change when you look at them through a sheet of glass? Notice how you feel and the thoughts that come to your mind watching through a sheet of glass as your client decides whether or not to circumcise their baby. (Allow 30–60 seconds to pass.)

Remove the glass and be there with your client as they discussing circumcision. They start to lean toward the decision to have their baby circumcised. Notice how hearing this feels for you. What thoughts begin to enter your mind? Take some moments to be with your thoughts and feelings. (Allow 30–60 seconds to pass.)

Place the sheet of glass back between you and your client as they seem to lean toward the decision to have their baby circumcised. Does having a sheet of glass between you change your thoughts or feelings? Again, take some time to be with your thoughts and feelings as you sit on the other side of a sheet of glass from your client discussing their desire to have their baby circumcised. (Allow 30–60 seconds to pass.)

Now, return to simply being with your client. simply be with them. There is no particular discussion happening. Simply be with them in your imagination and notice your thoughts and feelings. (Allow 30–60 seconds to pass.)

Again, the conversation moves to the topic of circumcision. Now they start to speak as though they will choose not to have their baby circumcised. Notice how it is for you to be with your client leaning towards opting not to have their baby circumcised. Be with your thoughts and feelings. (Allow 30–60 seconds to pass.)

And now, place a sheet of glass between you and your client again as they seem to lean toward the decision to not have their baby circumcised. Does having a sheet of glass between you change how you feel or the thoughts that arise in your mind? Again, take some time to be with your thoughts and feelings as you sit on the other side of a sheet of glass from your client as they discuss their desire to not have their baby circumcised. (Allow 30–60 seconds to pass.)

Finally, return to simply being in the room with your client. Be there in the room with them. Notice how you feel and whether your mind brings you to any of the above scenarios. Be there. Be with your thoughts and be with your feelings. (Allow 30–60 seconds to pass.)

3. Presence Yourself

Before you step away completely, take a moment to bring your awareness back into the present moment. Open your eyes and look around you. See what is in the space with you. Hear the sounds that are around you. Feel the air around you and the body you are living in. You can even pay attention to what you are tasting and smelling. Take some moments to bring your attention to the present moment and away from the topic you just explored.

4. Introspection

How was that for you?

What did you learn about yourself?

Did any of your reactions surprise you?

How will you bring the experience of working The Neutrality Exercise on this topic into your life?

The Neutrality Exercise Workbook for Birth Doulas

Topic 17: You Choose

1. A Basic Grounding

Bringing Attention to Your Breath

You can sit, stand, lie down, or do whatever works best for you. Our aim is to have your body in a state of balance, release, and maybe even in a state of pleasure. If you are seated, your weight should be evenly distributed on your sit bones. If you are standing, keep your weight evenly distributed between your feet. If you are pregnant and lying down, do so on your left side with pillows to support you. If you are not pregnant and want to lie down, do so on your back, perhaps with your knees up and feet on the ground if that is more comfortable for you. Aim for comfort. Aim for relaxation. Aim for pleasure.

Once you are settled, close your eyes or bring them to a soft gaze—whichever brings relaxation to your eyes.

Now, bring your attention to your breathing. Be a witness to it. Notice. Is it fast? Is it slow? Is it deep? Is it shallow? Witness your breathing body like you would calmly witness a new baby discovering its feet for the first time. simply be with it. Feel your inhales and exhales.

You can now become a bit more active with your breath. If you feel a desire to change your breathing at all—perhaps change its rhythm—please do. Maybe you notice you would like to take a deep breath in and let out a sigh. Maybe you feel like doing a little rapid breathing to free it up. Or maybe it's all good just how it is. simply take a moment to experiment with your breath.

Once you have made any desired changes, bring yourself back to the passive witness state again. Be with your breathing. Be with your body. Be with yourself.

Grounding the Body

Bring your attention deep into your lower abdomen, focusing simply in front of the spine at the core of your body. Imagine there is a cylindrical tube that attaches this point in your body to the surface of the Earth. You can imagine this tube to be whatever you choose: a hose, a root, a tree trunk, a lava tube, a ray of light. Really see it in your mind's eye and imagine it connecting the center of you with the Earth.

On your next exhale, imagine your tube sinking deeper into the Earth. It falls easily. It gets longer and longer. It falls through all the layers of the Earth. It falls through rock, water, and magma—all the way down to the very center of the Earth. Feel it as the core of your body firmly attaches to the core of Mother Earth. Your bottom is heavy and you feel your connection.

On your next exhale, imagine taking all the energy you don't need right now and sending it down through the tube. Give it to Mother Earth. You don't have to see it or know what it is, simply suggest to yourself that you're letting go of whatever isn't needed right now. It is falling toward the center of the Earth. Where there is tension or pain in your body, relax the area and let it all drain into Mother Earth. This is her compost; she will take it and turn it into fertile soil.

Try to match your breathing with your release: on your inhale, gather all your undesirable energy into a blob of goo and then on your exhale, let it drop down your tube into the Earth. Or you can be more physical about it. On your inhale, stand up and tense your muscles, bringing in and intensifying the energy, and then on your

exhale, release all your muscles and fall over or into your seat.

Take some time to practice this on your own for a bit, unguided. During this time, give whatever you want over to Mother Earth through your grounding cord.

Now, take a moment to stop your download and simply feel yourself, feel your grounding cord. Be with what is for a few moments. Bring your attention back to the room slowly. If your eyes are closed, open them slowly. Wiggle your body around a bit. Do what you need to do to bring your awareness back into the room and be present with the people who are here.

2. The Neutrality Exercise - Pick a topic and write it here:

Use one of the scripts below or write your own.

A. The Neutrality Exercise:

Imagine you are in the presence of your stated topic. Just be in a room with it. Notice how you feel being in a room with it. Be there and be with how you are feeling and the thoughts that come to your mind. (Allow 30-60secs to pass.)

Next, imagine there is a sheet of glass between you and your topic. Notice. Do your feelings change at all while you look at it through a piece of glass? DO your thoughts change? Notice how you feel and the thoughts that come to your mind being in the room with it while having a piece of glass between you and it. (Allow 30-60secs to pass.)

Now, image you are in a huge room - think of a ball room or large conference room. Imagine your topic is at the opposite end of the

room from you; you can see it, but from far away. Investigate how this feels and what thoughts arise. Did your reaction change at all from the prior scenarios. (Allow 30-60secs to pass.)

Now imagine you are at the top of a tall tower and the topic is outside the tower, down on the ground. You can barely see it but you know it is there. See what this feels like and what thoughts come to your mind. (Allow 30-60secs to pass.)

Finally, return to simply being with your topic. Be with your topic and be with how you feel and the thoughts that come to your mind. (Allow 30-60secs to pass.)

B. The Neutrality Exercise (Contrasting):

Imagine you are in the presence of your stated topic. Just be in a room with it. Notice how you feel being in a room with it. Be there and be with how you are feeling and the thoughts that come to your mind. (Allow 30-60secs to pass.)

Next, imagine there is a sheet of glass between you and your topic. Notice. Do your feelings change at all while you look at it through a piece of glass? Notice how you feel and the thoughts that come to your mind being in the room with it while having a piece of glass between you and it. (Allow 30-60secs to pass.)

Now, image you are in a huge room - think of a ball room or large conference room. Imagine your topic is at the opposite end of the room from you; you can see it, but from far away. Investigate how this feels and whether your feelings or thoughts change from the prior scenarios. (Allow 30-60secs to pass.)

Now, go back to just being your topic. Again, just be in its presence. Notice how you feel and what thoughts arise being there with it. Be

there and be with how you are. (Allow 30-60secs to pass.)

Next, imagine you are in the presence of a contrast to your stated topic. Just be in a room with it. Notice how you feel and the thoughts that come to your mind being in a room with it. Be there and be with how you are. (Allow 30-60secs to pass.)

And then imagine there is a sheet of glass between you and the contrast to your topic. Notice. Do your feelings or thoughts change when you look at it through a piece of glass? Notice how you feel and the thoughts that come to your mind being in the room with it while having a piece of glass between you and it. (Allow 30-60secs to pass.)

Now, image you are in a huge room. Imagine you are at the opposite end of this large room from your contrasting topic; you can see it, but from far away. Investigate how this is for you and whether your thoughts or feelings change from the prior scenarios. (Allow 30-60secs to pass.)

Finally, go back to just being your topic. Again, just be in its presence. Maybe notice if your imagination comes to rest more on the original topic or the contrast to it. Notice how you feel and the thoughts that come to your mind being there with whichever you find. Be there and be with how you are. (Allow 30-60secs to pass.)

3. Presence Yourself

Before you step away completely, take a moment to bring your awareness back into the present moment. Open your eyes and look around you. See what is in the space with you. Hear the sounds that are around you. Feel the air around you and the body you are living in. You can even pay attention to what you are tasting and smelling.

Take some moments to bring your attention to the present moment and away from the topic you just explored.

4. Introspection

How was that for you?

What did you learn about yourself?

Did any of your reactions surprise you?

How will you bring the experience of working The Neutrality Exercise on this topic into your life?

Topic 18: You Choose

1. A Basic Grounding

Bringing Attention to Your Breath

You can sit, stand, lie down, or do whatever works best for you. Our aim is to have your body in a state of balance, release, and maybe even in a state of pleasure. If you are seated, your weight should be evenly distributed on your sit bones. If you are standing, keep your weight evenly distributed between your feet. If you are pregnant and lying down, do so on your left side with pillows to support you. If you are not pregnant and want to lie down, do so on your back, perhaps with your knees up and feet on the ground if that is more comfortable for you. Aim for comfort. Aim for relaxation. Aim for pleasure.

Once you are settled, close your eyes or bring them to a soft gaze—whichever brings relaxation to your eyes.

Now, bring your attention to your breathing. Be a witness to it. Notice. Is it fast? Is it slow? Is it deep? Is it shallow? Witness your breathing body like you would calmly witness a new baby discovering its feet for the first time. simply be with it. Feel your inhales and exhales.

You can now become a bit more active with your breath. If you feel a desire to change your breathing at all—perhaps change its rhythm—please do. Maybe you notice you would like to take a deep breath in and let out a sigh. Maybe you feel like doing a little rapid breathing to free it up. Or maybe it's all good just how it is. simply take a moment to experiment with your breath.

Once you have made any desired changes, bring yourself back to the passive witness state again. Be with your breathing. Be with your body. Be with yourself.

Grounding the Body

Bring your attention deep into your lower abdomen, focusing simply in front of the spine at the core of your body. Imagine there is a cylindrical tube that attaches this point in your body to the surface of the Earth. You can imagine this tube to be whatever you choose: a hose, a root, a tree trunk, a lava tube, a ray of light. Really see it in your mind's eye and imagine it connecting the center of you with the Earth.

On your next exhale, imagine your tube sinking deeper into the Earth. It falls easily. It gets longer and longer. It falls through all the layers of the Earth. It falls through rock, water, and magma—all the way down to the very center of the Earth. Feel it as the core of your body firmly attaches to the core of Mother Earth. Your bottom is heavy and you feel your connection.

On your next exhale, imagine taking all the energy you don't need right now and sending it down through the tube. Give it to Mother Earth. You don't have to see it or know what it is, simply suggest to yourself that you're letting go of whatever isn't needed right now. It is falling toward the center of the Earth. Where there is tension or pain in your body, relax the area and let it all drain into Mother Earth. This is her compost; she will take it and turn it into fertile soil.

Try to match your breathing with your release: on your inhale, gather all your undesirable energy into a blob of goo and then on your exhale, let it drop down your tube into the Earth. Or you can be more physical about it. On your inhale, stand up and tense your muscles, bringing in and intensifying the energy, and then on your

exhale, release all your muscles and fall over or into your seat.

Take some time to practice this on your own for a bit, unguided. During this time, give whatever you want over to Mother Earth through your grounding cord.

Now, take a moment to stop your download and simply feel yourself, feel your grounding cord. Be with what is for a few moments. Bring your attention back to the room slowly. If your eyes are closed, open them slowly. Wiggle your body around a bit. Do what you need to do to bring your awareness back into the room and be present with the people who are here.

2. The Neutrality Exercise - Pick a topic and write it here:

Use one of the scripts below or write your own.

A. The Neutrality Exercise:

Imagine you are in the presence of your stated topic. Just be in a room with it. Notice how you feel being in a room with it. Be there and be with how you are feeling and the thoughts that come to your mind. (Allow 30-60secs to pass.)

Next, imagine there is a sheet of glass between you and your topic. Notice. Do your feelings change at all while you look at it through a piece of glass? DO your thoughts change? Notice how you feel and the thoughts that come to your mind being in the room with it while having a piece of glass between you and it. (Allow 30-60secs to pass.)

Now, image you are in a huge room - think of a ball room or large conference room. Imagine your topic is at the opposite end of the

room from you; you can see it, but from far away. Investigate how this feels and what thoughts arise. Did your reaction change at all from the prior scenarios. (Allow 30-60secs to pass.)

Now imagine you are at the top of a tall tower and the topic is outside the tower, down on the ground. You can barely see it but you know it is there. See what this feels like and what thoughts come to your mind. (Allow 30-60secs to pass.)

Finally, return to simply being with your topic. Be with your topic and be with how you feel and the thoughts that come to your mind. (Allow 30-60secs to pass.)

B. The Neutrality Exercise (Contrasting):

Imagine you are in the presence of your stated topic. Just be in a room with it. Notice how you feel being in a room with it. Be there and be with how you are feeling and the thoughts that come to your mind. (Allow 30-60secs to pass.)

Next, imagine there is a sheet of glass between you and your topic. Notice. Do your feelings change at all while you look at it through a piece of glass? Notice how you feel and the thoughts that come to your mind being in the room with it while having a piece of glass between you and it. (Allow 30-60secs to pass.)

Now, image you are in a huge room - think of a ball room or large conference room. Imagine your topic is at the opposite end of the room from you; you can see it, but from far away. Investigate how this feels and whether your feelings or thoughts change from the prior scenarios. (Allow 30-60secs to pass.)

Now, go back to just being your topic. Again, just be in its presence. Notice how you feel and what thoughts arise being there with it. Be

there and be with how you are. (Allow 30-60secs to pass.)

Next, imagine you are in the presence of a contrast to your stated topic. Just be in a room with it. Notice how you feel and the thoughts that come to your mind being in a room with it. Be there and be with how you are. (Allow 30-60secs to pass.)

And then imagine there is a sheet of glass between you and the contrast to your topic. Notice. Do your feelings or thoughts change when you look at it through a piece of glass? Notice how you feel and the thoughts that come to your mind being in the room with it while having a piece of glass between you and it. (Allow 30-60secs to pass.)

Now, image you are in a huge room. Imagine you are at the opposite end of this large room from your contrasting topic; you can see it, but from far away. Investigate how this is for you and whether your thoughts or feelings change from the prior scenarios. (Allow 30-60secs to pass.)

Finally, go back to just being your topic. Again, just be in its presence. Maybe notice if your imagination comes to rest more on the original topic or the contrast to it. Notice how you feel and the thoughts that come to your mind being there with whichever you find. Be there and be with how you are. (Allow 30-60secs to pass.)

3. Presence Yourself

Before you step away completely, take a moment to bring your awareness back into the present moment. Open your eyes and look around you. See what is in the space with you. Hear the sounds that are around you. Feel the air around you and the body you are living in. You can even pay attention to what you are tasting and smelling.

Take some moments to bring your attention to the present moment and away from the topic you just explored.

4. Introspection

How was that for you?

What did you learn about yourself?

Did any of your reactions surprise you?

How will you bring the experience of working The Neutrality Exercise on this topic into your life?

The Neutrality Exercise Workbook for Birth Doulas

Topic 19: You Choose

1. A Basic Grounding

Bringing Attention to Your Breath

You can sit, stand, lie down, or do whatever works best for you. Our aim is to have your body in a state of balance, release, and maybe even in a state of pleasure. If you are seated, your weight should be evenly distributed on your sit bones. If you are standing, keep your weight evenly distributed between your feet. If you are pregnant and lying down, do so on your left side with pillows to support you. If you are not pregnant and want to lie down, do so on your back, perhaps with your knees up and feet on the ground if that is more comfortable for you. Aim for comfort. Aim for relaxation. Aim for pleasure.

Once you are settled, close your eyes or bring them to a soft gaze—whichever brings relaxation to your eyes.

Now, bring your attention to your breathing. Be a witness to it. Notice. Is it fast? Is it slow? Is it deep? Is it shallow? Witness your breathing body like you would calmly witness a new baby discovering its feet for the first time. simply be with it. Feel your inhales and exhales.

You can now become a bit more active with your breath. If you feel a desire to change your breathing at all—perhaps change its rhythm—please do. Maybe you notice you would like to take a deep breath in and let out a sigh. Maybe you feel like doing a little rapid breathing to free it up. Or maybe it's all good just how it is. simply take a moment to experiment with your breath.

Once you have made any desired changes, bring yourself back to the passive witness state again. Be with your breathing. Be with your body. Be with yourself.

Grounding the Body

Bring your attention deep into your lower abdomen, focusing simply in front of the spine at the core of your body. Imagine there is a cylindrical tube that attaches this point in your body to the surface of the Earth. You can imagine this tube to be whatever you choose: a hose, a root, a tree trunk, a lava tube, a ray of light. Really see it in your mind's eye and imagine it connecting the center of you with the Earth.

On your next exhale, imagine your tube sinking deeper into the Earth. It falls easily. It gets longer and longer. It falls through all the layers of the Earth. It falls through rock, water, and magma—all the way down to the very center of the Earth. Feel it as the core of your body firmly attaches to the core of Mother Earth. Your bottom is heavy and you feel your connection.

On your next exhale, imagine taking all the energy you don't need right now and sending it down through the tube. Give it to Mother Earth. You don't have to see it or know what it is, simply suggest to yourself that you're letting go of whatever isn't needed right now. It is falling toward the center of the Earth. Where there is tension or pain in your body, relax the area and let it all drain into Mother Earth. This is her compost; she will take it and turn it into fertile soil.

Try to match your breathing with your release: on your inhale, gather all your undesirable energy into a blob of goo and then on your exhale, let it drop down your tube into the Earth. Or you can be more physical about it. On your inhale, stand up and tense your muscles, bringing in and intensifying the energy, and then on your

exhale, release all your muscles and fall over or into your seat.

Take some time to practice this on your own for a bit, unguided. During this time, give whatever you want over to Mother Earth through your grounding cord.

Now, take a moment to stop your download and simply feel yourself, feel your grounding cord. Be with what is for a few moments. Bring your attention back to the room slowly. If your eyes are closed, open them slowly. Wiggle your body around a bit. Do what you need to do to bring your awareness back into the room and be present with the people who are here.

2. The Neutrality Exercise - Pick a topic and write it here:

Use one of the scripts below or write your own.

A. The Neutrality Exercise:

Imagine you are in the presence of your stated topic. Just be in a room with it. Notice how you feel being in a room with it. Be there and be with how you are feeling and the thoughts that come to your mind. (Allow 30-60secs to pass.)

Next, imagine there is a sheet of glass between you and your topic. Notice. Do your feelings change at all while you look at it through a piece of glass? DO your thoughts change? Notice how you feel and the thoughts that come to your mind being in the room with it while having a piece of glass between you and it. (Allow 30-60secs to pass.)

Now, image you are in a huge room - think of a ball room or large conference room. Imagine your topic is at the opposite end of the

room from you; you can see it, but from far away. Investigate how this feels and what thoughts arise. Did your reaction change at all from the prior scenarios. (Allow 30-60secs to pass.)

Now imagine you are at the top of a tall tower and the topic is outside the tower, down on the ground. You can barely see it but you know it is there. See what this feels like and what thoughts come to your mind. (Allow 30-60secs to pass.)

Finally, return to simply being with your topic. Be with your topic and be with how you feel and the thoughts that come to your mind. (Allow 30-60secs to pass.)

B. The Neutrality Exercise (Contrasting):

Imagine you are in the presence of your stated topic. Just be in a room with it. Notice how you feel being in a room with it. Be there and be with how you are feeling and the thoughts that come to your mind. (Allow 30-60secs to pass.)

Next, imagine there is a sheet of glass between you and your topic. Notice. Do your feelings change at all while you look at it through a piece of glass? Notice how you feel and the thoughts that come to your mind being in the room with it while having a piece of glass between you and it. (Allow 30-60secs to pass.)

Now, image you are in a huge room - think of a ball room or large conference room. Imagine your topic is at the opposite end of the room from you; you can see it, but from far away. Investigate how this feels and whether your feelings or thoughts change from the prior scenarios. (Allow 30-60secs to pass.)

Now, go back to just being your topic. Again, just be in its presence. Notice how you feel and what thoughts arise being there with it. Be

there and be with how you are. (Allow 30-60secs to pass.)

Next, imagine you are in the presence of a contrast to your stated topic. Just be in a room with it. Notice how you feel and the thoughts that come to your mind being in a room with it. Be there and be with how you are. (Allow 30-60secs to pass.)

And then imagine there is a sheet of glass between you and the contrast to your topic. Notice. Do your feelings or thoughts change when you look at it through a piece of glass? Notice how you feel and the thoughts that come to your mind being in the room with it while having a piece of glass between you and it. (Allow 30-60secs to pass.)

Now, image you are in a huge room. Imagine you are at the opposite end of this large room from your contrasting topic; you can see it, but from far away. Investigate how this is for you and whether your thoughts or feelings change from the prior scenarios. (Allow 30-60secs to pass.)

Finally, go back to just being your topic. Again, just be in its presence. Maybe notice if your imagination comes to rest more on the original topic or the contrast to it. Notice how you feel and the thoughts that come to your mind being there with whichever you find. Be there and be with how you are. (Allow 30-60secs to pass.)

3. Presence Yourself

Before you step away completely, take a moment to bring your awareness back into the present moment. Open your eyes and look around you. See what is in the space with you. Hear the sounds that are around you. Feel the air around you and the body you are living in. You can even pay attention to what you are tasting and smelling.

Take some moments to bring your attention to the present moment and away from the topic you just explored.

4. Introspection

How was that for you?

What did you learn about yourself?

Did any of your reactions surprise you?

How will you bring the experience of working The Neutrality Exercise on this topic into your life?

Topic 20: You Choose

1. A Basic Grounding

Bringing Attention to Your Breath

You can sit, stand, lie down, or do whatever works best for you. Our aim is to have your body in a state of balance, release, and maybe even in a state of pleasure. If you are seated, your weight should be evenly distributed on your sit bones. If you are standing, keep your weight evenly distributed between your feet. If you are pregnant and lying down, do so on your left side with pillows to support you. If you are not pregnant and want to lie down, do so on your back, perhaps with your knees up and feet on the ground if that is more comfortable for you. Aim for comfort. Aim for relaxation. Aim for pleasure.

Once you are settled, close your eyes or bring them to a soft gaze—whichever brings relaxation to your eyes.

Now, bring your attention to your breathing. Be a witness to it. Notice. Is it fast? Is it slow? Is it deep? Is it shallow? Witness your breathing body like you would calmly witness a new baby discovering its feet for the first time. simply be with it. Feel your inhales and exhales.

You can now become a bit more active with your breath. If you feel a desire to change your breathing at all—perhaps change its rhythm—please do. Maybe you notice you would like to take a deep breath in and let out a sigh. Maybe you feel like doing a little rapid breathing to free it up. Or maybe it's all good just how it is. simply take a moment to experiment with your breath.

Once you have made any desired changes, bring yourself back to the passive witness state again. Be with your breathing. Be with your body. Be with yourself.

Grounding the Body

Bring your attention deep into your lower abdomen, focusing simply in front of the spine at the core of your body. Imagine there is a cylindrical tube that attaches this point in your body to the surface of the Earth. You can imagine this tube to be whatever you choose: a hose, a root, a tree trunk, a lava tube, a ray of light. Really see it in your mind's eye and imagine it connecting the center of you with the Earth.

On your next exhale, imagine your tube sinking deeper into the Earth. It falls easily. It gets longer and longer. It falls through all the layers of the Earth. It falls through rock, water, and magma—all the way down to the very center of the Earth. Feel it as the core of your body firmly attaches to the core of Mother Earth. Your bottom is heavy and you feel your connection.

On your next exhale, imagine taking all the energy you don't need right now and sending it down through the tube. Give it to Mother Earth. You don't have to see it or know what it is, simply suggest to yourself that you're letting go of whatever isn't needed right now. It is falling toward the center of the Earth. Where there is tension or pain in your body, relax the area and let it all drain into Mother Earth. This is her compost; she will take it and turn it into fertile soil.

Try to match your breathing with your release: on your inhale, gather all your undesirable energy into a blob of goo and then on your exhale, let it drop down your tube into the Earth. Or you can be more physical about it. On your inhale, stand up and tense your muscles, bringing in and intensifying the energy, and then on your

exhale, release all your muscles and fall over or into your seat.

Take some time to practice this on your own for a bit, unguided. During this time, give whatever you want over to Mother Earth through your grounding cord.

Now, take a moment to stop your download and simply feel yourself, feel your grounding cord. Be with what is for a few moments. Bring your attention back to the room slowly. If your eyes are closed, open them slowly. Wiggle your body around a bit. Do what you need to do to bring your awareness back into the room and be present with the people who are here.

2. The Neutrality Exercise - Pick a topic and write it here:

Use one of the scripts below or write your own.

A. The Neutrality Exercise:

Imagine you are in the presence of your stated topic. Just be in a room with it. Notice how you feel being in a room with it. Be there and be with how you are feeling and the thoughts that come to your mind. (Allow 30-60secs to pass.)

Next, imagine there is a sheet of glass between you and your topic. Notice. Do your feelings change at all while you look at it through a piece of glass? DO your thoughts change? Notice how you feel and the thoughts that come to your mind being in the room with it while having a piece of glass between you and it. (Allow 30-60secs to pass.)

Now, image you are in a huge room - think of a ball room or large conference room. Imagine your topic is at the opposite end of the

room from you; you can see it, but from far away. Investigate how this feels and what thoughts arise. Did your reaction change at all from the prior scenarios. (Allow 30-60secs to pass.)

Now imagine you are at the top of a tall tower and the topic is outside the tower, down on the ground. You can barely see it but you know it is there. See what this feels like and what thoughts come to your mind. (Allow 30-60secs to pass.)

Finally, return to simply being with your topic. Be with your topic and be with how you feel and the thoughts that come to your mind. (Allow 30-60secs to pass.)

B. The Neutrality Exercise (Contrasting):

Imagine you are in the presence of your stated topic. Just be in a room with it. Notice how you feel being in a room with it. Be there and be with how you are feeling and the thoughts that come to your mind. (Allow 30-60secs to pass.)

Next, imagine there is a sheet of glass between you and your topic. Notice. Do your feelings change at all while you look at it through a piece of glass? Notice how you feel and the thoughts that come to your mind being in the room with it while having a piece of glass between you and it. (Allow 30-60secs to pass.)

Now, image you are in a huge room - think of a ball room or large conference room. Imagine your topic is at the opposite end of the room from you; you can see it, but from far away. Investigate how this feels and whether your feelings or thoughts change from the prior scenarios. (Allow 30-60secs to pass.)

Now, go back to just being your topic. Again, just be in its presence. Notice how you feel and what thoughts arise being there with it. Be

there and be with how you are. (Allow 30-60secs to pass.)

Next, imagine you are in the presence of a contrast to your stated topic. Just be in a room with it. Notice how you feel and the thoughts that come to your mind being in a room with it. Be there and be with how you are. (Allow 30-60secs to pass.)

And then imagine there is a sheet of glass between you and the contrast to your topic. Notice. Do your feelings or thoughts change when you look at it through a piece of glass? Notice how you feel and the thoughts that come to your mind being in the room with it while having a piece of glass between you and it. (Allow 30-60secs to pass.)

Now, image you are in a huge room. Imagine you are at the opposite end of this large room from your contrasting topic; you can see it, but from far away. Investigate how this is for you and whether your thoughts or feelings change from the prior scenarios. (Allow 30-60secs to pass.)

Finally, go back to just being your topic. Again, just be in its presence. Maybe notice if your imagination comes to rest more on the original topic or the contrast to it. Notice how you feel and the thoughts that come to your mind being there with whichever you find. Be there and be with how you are. (Allow 30-60secs to pass.)

3. Presence Yourself

Before you step away completely, take a moment to bring your awareness back into the present moment. Open your eyes and look around you. See what is in the space with you. Hear the sounds that are around you. Feel the air around you and the body you are living in. You can even pay attention to what you are tasting and smelling.

Take some moments to bring your attention to the present moment and away from the topic you just explored.

4. Introspection

How was that for you?

What did you learn about yourself?

Did any of your reactions surprise you?

How will you bring the experience of working The Neutrality Exercise on this topic into your life?

Bonus Practice: Analyzing Bias

Now that you have completed this workbook, take some moments to ponder bias as it relates to The Neutrality Exercise.

Do you feel like doing The Neutrality Exercise has helped you to see your own biases better?

How is it for you to think about your biases?

Do you believe The Neutrality Exercise will change anything about how you show up in the world?

Thank you!

We too have done this work. For that reason, we know how challenging it can be.

We also know the potential we can harness together when we all do this kind of work.

Thank you from us to you for being willing to use your time and attention to become just that much more aware of who you are.

If you are interested in doing more, visit www.holisticpeercounseling.com.

A Note From The Author

I am not the creator of The Neutrality Exercise. In truth, I am unsure of who is. It was first brought to my attention by Kristen Rawson in their version of Holistic Peer Counseling which they called Holistic Peer Support. Likewise, the concept of grounding to the center of the earth is not my brain child. This idea has roots in many traditions and was first brought into my awareness by Teri Ciacchi.

All of that said, it is through the countless hours of Siddha Yoga devotional practice I partook in as a child that I learned the power of meditative practice. I bring that experience to this book and these practices.

Likewise, it is my mother, Kathryn Julia who made the point of raising me in the world of embodiment. It is through embodiment that she continues to find healing and recovery from the violent abuse of her childhood. Learning to live IN her body has brought her recovery. As such, she raised me to use my own body as a medium for empowerment and healing. I bring these tools to this book, as well.

Finally, a big thank you to my husband, my children and those who work with me. Each of you continues to help me and my work evolve. I love you all <3.

www.ingramcontent.com/pod-product-compliance
Lightning Source LLC
Chambersburg PA
CBHW071310220526
45468CB00001B/323